What readers are saying about
FROM MOUNTAINS TO MEDICINE

From Mountains to Medicine is the story of Dr. Erica Elliott's magical journey off the beaten path. The utter exuberance she has for life is contagious. An intrepid explorer of cultures, people, mountains, and medicine, Erica's dedication to making people's lives better is the golden thread that holds her world together. A physician of expansive vision and skill, "La Cabra Montés" (the mountain goat), as she was named after scaling the highest peak in the Western Hemisphere, ultimately became "The Health Detective." The story of that unlikely transformation ignites the imagination and opens the heart. This is a book you'll want to share with all the people you love.

—JOAN BORYSENKO, PHD
speaker and *New York Times* best-selling
author of *Minding the Body, Mending the Mind*

Erica Elliott is a natural-born storyteller. Her deeply affecting memoir is about family and the essential journey of self-discovery she went on to find her soul's purpose. This book takes you on a wild, world odyssey through the Swiss Alps, the Peace Corps in Ecuador, and mountain climbing in Argentina. Elliott's writing is honest and intoxicating; she writes about diverse Indigenous people, culture, and communities around the world in an intimate, visceral way. Ultimately, Elliott's wise heart leads her home to discover what was there all along—her destiny to be a healer.

—DEBRA ROSENMAN
author/editor of the multi-award-winning book
*The Chimpanzee Chronicles: Stories of
Heartbreak and Hope from Behind the Bars*

From Mountains to Medicine: Scaling the Heights in Search of My Calling is a truly compelling, fascinating, and engaging journey—actually many journeys of Erica Elliott's life. I found myself laughing out loud, holding my breath, opening my eyes wide in shock, at times exclaiming "holy sh*t!"—and I imagine you will too. It is much more than a memoir. It is so engrossing I forgot I was reading a book, and I look forward to the day when it is made into a movie. Erica's writing is clear and straightforward, taking you step by step through pivotal moments in her life, as if you were traveling right along with her. Definitely a must-read!

—ALAN QUESTEL
author of *Practice Intentional Acts of Kindness*

In this mind-bending and heart-opening memoir, Erica Elliott takes us on the intimate journey of finding her ultimate purpose in life. Each of us is offered clues in our lives, at first as quiet as a tiny mountain spring, which, if we listen and follow, can become a river plunging toward the sea. The miracle of the rites of passage that Erica offers here is her listening and following, her opening awareness and courage along the way, and her remarkable ability to bring us along. In our taking this journey with her, we, too, can become more attentive and devoted to saying "Yes!" to the opportunities that life affords us.

—HEIDI SPARKES GUBER
co-author of *A Whole Greater than Its Parts: Exploring the Role of Emergence in Complex Social Change*

In a voice that always cuts to the heart of things, Erica Elliott describes her adventures in mountaineering and the Peace Corps in the Andes in colorful, imagistic word paintings. She also looks back on her life in a large itinerant army family, and how she overcame its difficult emotional legacy. All this prepares her for a life healing others. Her inspiring story and heartfelt voice have their own curative properties.

—SALLY ABBOTT
author of *Miami in Virgo*

Right from the beginning of her story, [Erica Elliott] draws the reader into her narrative as she threads her way through the turbulent early years of her life, overcoming many challenges along the way. Her guiding star is her search for meaning and purpose, which leads her to some spellbinding adventures... [You] will find this book uplifting, inspiring, and full of wisdom.

—ALICE K. LADAS, EDD
author of the *New York Times* bestseller
The G Spot and Other Discoveries About Human Sexuality

A person's purpose in life seems to live in that sweet spot where your deepest joy intersects with your unique skill set and also with the world's endless need. It is a treat and an education to follow the young, courageous, and tenacious Erica Elliott through her extraordinary journey as she puts together all three. Full of insight as well as cultural and mountaineering adventure, *From Mountains to Medicine* is a great read.

—CHRIS HOFFMAN
author of *The Hoop and the Tree: A Compass for Finding a Deeper Relationship with All Life*

Few coming-of-age tales carry a reader so deeply into the heart and soul of the one who lived it. Dr. Erica Merriam Elliott takes us through her acutely intimate and profoundly explicit struggles to find her own unique purpose and meanings in life, work, and vocation... The reader will find breathtaking moments of sheer terror and the power of her unfathomable tenacity and courage in the midst of astonishing beauty and in the face of bone-crushing poverty. *From Mountains to Medicine,* the second in her memoir trilogy, is a story of resilience, giving us remarkable insight into what makes us supremely human and what drives us to finding our distinctive path in life... Erica shines a bright light on the multiple possibilities of what it means to be whole, to be human, and to be hopeful. Your time and energy in following her saga will bring you to tears and shouts of delight.

—THE REVEREND CANON TED KARPF
Episcopal priest and author of *Acts of Forgiveness: Faith Journeys of a Gay Priest* and principal editor of the World Health Organization's *Restoring Hope: Decent Care in the Midst of HIV/AIDS*

ALSO BY ERICA M. ELLIOTT

Medicine and Miracles in the High Desert: My Life Among the Navajo People
  Bear & Company/Inner Traditions

Prescriptions for a Healthy House, 3rd ed.
  Co-author, with Paula Baker-Laporte and John Banta
  New Society Press

Ñucunchimunda
  bilingual storybook in Quechua and Spanish
  Instituto Interandino de Desarollo

FROM MOUNTAINS TO MEDICINE

Scaling the Heights in Search of My Calling

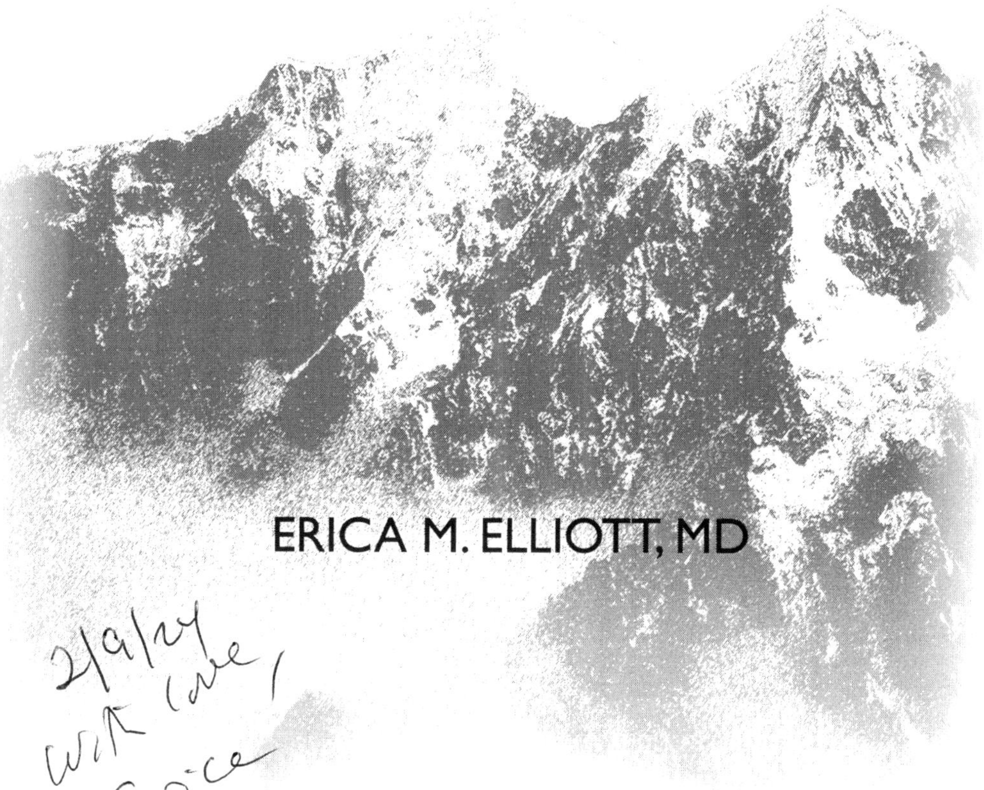

ERICA M. ELLIOTT, MD

2/9/24
With love,
Erica

FOREWORD BY LARRY DOSSEY, MD

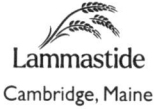

Lammastide
Cambridge, Maine

© 2023 by Erica M. Elliott
All Rights Reserved.

No part of this book may be reproduced or transmitted in any form or by any means, graphic, electronic or mechanical, including photocopying, recording, taping or by any information storage or retrieval system, without the written permission of the publisher, except for brief passages used in a review.

Library of Congress Cataloging-in-Publication Data

Elliott, Erica M., author.
From Mountains to Medicine / by Erica M. Elliott.

ISBN: 979-8-9876200-0-7
Library of Congress Control Number: 2023916329

1. Memoir 2. Mountaineering 3. Medicine

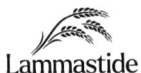
Lammastide

Published by Lammastide
946 Dexter Road
Cambridge, Maine 04923
www.lammastide.com

Lammastide is a division of Demeter, LLC

Book design by Kathleen Dexter – KDInkandImage.net

Cover images
   Mountains: pexels.com/pexels-trixiella-lichtenberg-666010
   Erica and tent: Unknown photographer, circa 1975

This book is dedicated to all my climbing friends
in the Club de Andinismo Politécnica who
took me under their wings and welcomed me
into their world of climbing.

Les doy a todos un gran abrazo montañero.

CONTENTS

i	Foreword by Larry Dossey, MD
iii	Note to the Reader
1	Chapter 1 · How Did I Get Here?
4	Chapter 2 · First Day of College
13	Chapter 3 · My New Life
18	Chapter 4 · Marriage
26	Chapter 5 · Breakdown
32	Chapter 6 · Archeology of the Soul
36	Chapter 7 · My Father and Me
42	Chapter 8 · At the Pub
49	Chapter 9 · Cutting the Braid
55	Chapter 10 · Cutting Loose
58	Chapter 11 · Jean Pierre
67	Chapter 12 · Slaying the Dragons
73	Chapter 13 · My Mother and Me
83	Chapter 14 · Breakthrough
86	Chapter 15 · Wrapping Up
91	Chapter 16 · Uncle Ernst
116	Chapter 17 · Peace Corps
129	Chapter 18 · Home Gardens
137	Chapter 19 · On the Ridge

146	Chapter 20 · Finding My Place High in the Andes
164	Chapter 21 · My Friend Mateo
175	Chapter 22 · From Paradise to Revolution
187	Chapter 23 · An Unplanned Event
195	Chapter 24 · La Compañía
207	Chapter 25 · Aconcagua—The Roof of the Americas
217	Chapter 26 · Getting Close
231	Chapter 27 · The Return
242	Chapter 28 · The View from the Top
255	Chapter 29 · On the Road
263	Chapter 30 · Back Home
269	Chapter 31 · Outward Bound
297	Chapter 32 · Buried Alive
303	Chapter 33 · Stanford Interview
315	Epilogue
319	Afterword
321	About the Author

FOREWORD
by Larry Dossey, MD

I first met Erica Elliott when I moved to Santa Fe, New Mexico, with my wife, Barbara, an author and pioneer in holistic nursing, following retirement from my internal medicine practice in Dallas, Texas. Erica was also a physician. Our friendship was a natural connection from the start.

As you will read in this captivating, mesmerizing account, Erica's journey has involved serial oscillations between life, death, and survival. Long after meeting her, I had no idea of the depth of her earlier gripping experiences. She is perhaps the most modest individual I have ever encountered, as evidenced by the way she so thoroughly under-expressed her harrowing history prior to this revealing book.

Besides our common profession, our similar histories no doubt made possible an unspoken connection between Erica and me. My earlier experience as a field battalion surgeon during the Vietnam War also involved many close calls. Somehow, we both managed to survive.

There is a folk saying: "Life breaks everyone. Many grow stronger at the broken places." Erica Elliott's memoir is compelling evidence for the truth of this adage. It is a resounding, powerful, and beautiful testament to the resilience of the human spirit against great odds.

This account holds nothing back. It records fragility and power, weakness and strength. It is the story of a unique, courageous woman who grew stronger at the broken places. It is a lesson for everyone.

Larry Dossey, MD

former chief of staff of Medical City Dallas Hospital and author of many books, including *Space, Time, & Medicine; Healing Words* (a *New York Times* bestseller), and *One Mind: How Your Individual Mind Is Part of a Greater Consciousness and Why It Matters*

NOTE TO THE READER

EVEN AS A CHILD, I sensed that I had a specific purpose in life—but I had no idea what that purpose was or how to go about finding it. In college, I realized that I would not be able to find my life's calling until I had found my true authentic self—which turned out to be quite different from the person I thought I was.

I begin telling my story by taking the reader along on the first of many harrowing snow and ice climbs I did while serving in the Peace Corps high in the Andes Mountains. As I navigated the steep, glaciated, and heavily crevassed slope, I asked myself why I felt such a strong pull to climb these perilous mountains. The answer to that question lay in the events that had occurred many years before that climb.

After the opening chapter, I bring the reader back in time to my college days. During my sophomore year, I lost my way and fell into an existential depression. The self I had known throughout my turbulent childhood fell apart. A gifted psychiatrist helped me turn this painful breakdown into an unimaginable blessing. Under his guidance, I began to dig into the archeology of my soul and made some life-changing and life-saving discoveries. I unearthed a more authentic version of myself—free from the myths and misperceptions I grew up with, and free from society's limiting beliefs about what was possible.

After graduating from college, I dove headlong into my future and began an almost mythological journey in search of meaning and purpose. Every life-changing experience I had along the way enriched me and helped to prepare me for finding and fulfilling my ultimate destiny.

While on my nearly decade-long search, I came to recognize that I had some innate gifts and talents that came naturally to me. When I dedicated these strengths I had to serving others in a meaningful way that enhanced their lives, I experienced immense joy and a sense of fulfillment.

In writing my story, I gave several of the main characters fictitious names to protect their privacy and, for the same reason, did not include photos that would reveal their identities. Some of the people have passed on—but quite a few are still in touch with me after all these years.

As a busy physician, I'm often tired at the end of a full day treating patients. But as I sit down to write in the evening, a burst of energy ignites in me when I think that my story might inspire others to find their passion and fearlessly pursue the longings of their soul.

Erica Elliott, MD
January 2024
Santa Fe, New Mexico

Chapter 1

HOW DID I GET HERE?

Ecuador, 1974

THE CREVASSES ON COTOPAXI IN ECUADOR, one of the highest active volcanoes in the world, continued all the way to the summit. Extreme exhaustion and the hypoxia that comes with high altitude made me want to doze off while climbing, but the fear of falling into a crevasse kept me awake through sheer force of will.

The first part of the climb involved zigzagging up the slope on the switchbacks. Our group—nine men and me—trudged along in silence, each of us alone in thought. I looked back at the chain of little bobbing lights moving steadily up the mountain in the blackness of night. We had begun our climb just after midnight in the freezing cold to take advantage of the hard-packed snow. We aimed to reach the summit by dawn.

Eventually the switchbacks ended, as our team faced terrain so steep we had to use our ice axes to maintain our balance. With every few steps, we swung the picks of our axes into the icy snow above our heads to prevent ourselves from falling backwards. Jorge, my friend and mountaineering mentor, showed me how to kick the hard-packed snow with my boots to make a little ledge with each step so I could transfer weight from one foot to the other without losing my footing and sliding down the mountain. Having to focus so intensely on each step kept me from becoming paralyzed with the fear of falling to my certain death.

The men had warned me about the many crevasses that we would traverse on the glacier and how careful we had to be so as not to fall into one of them. The first crevasse we passed had a wide, gaping mouth, making it easy to spot.

With Jorge's headlamp illuminating the area before me, I peered down into what looked like a bottomless expanse. A cold chill of fright ran up my spine. We found a way around the crevasse, carefully avoiding the precarious snow bridges that connected both sides. Jorge did not have to explain to me that the snow bridges could easily collapse under our weight.

My fear and excitement caused a burst of adrenaline that allowed me to remain alert and to keep up the pace that Jorge had set. After two or three hours, I began to pant while my heart pounded furiously in my chest. Reluctantly, I told Jorge I needed to stop and rest. He said we had to keep moving to reach the summit before the sun rose high enough to warm the snow, making it slushy.

As I leaned on my ice axe for support, gasping for air, Jorge offered a valuable climbing tip. He said that if I got into a set rhythm, putting one foot in front of the other, at a pace I could sustain, then I wouldn't need to rest. He said that resting would make the climb more difficult. I agreed to follow his advice.

Jorge set a slower pace for me, which meant that the other climbers in our group gradually passed us. I began silently counting my steps, "one and two and…" up to ten, then repeating the sequence over and over to maintain a rhythm that kept my mind focused.

The hours rolled by. I was in an altered state, as though hypnotized and detached from my body, perhaps from the low level of oxygen in my blood.

About halfway to the summit, ghostly, phantasmagoric shapes nearby jolted me into the present moment. Jorge had told me about these blocks of glacial ice formations, called *seracs*. Some looked like towers, while others had grown to the size of small houses. They appear where two crevasses intersect on the glacier and form an icefall.

Seracs can be dangerous to mountaineers because they have the potential to fall over without warning. In fact, the route to the summit is called *Rompe Corazones*, "Heart Breaker." I wondered what exactly "heart breaker" meant in this particular case. Did it mean that people die on this route and break their loved ones' hearts? Or that people had heart attacks on this route because it's so difficult? My brain was too oxygen-starved to puzzle it out, and by this time, I had developed an intense headache.

> *Why have I put myself in this precarious situation? Why in the world do I want to climb these mountains so badly? What is the point of all this? Am I going to get out of here alive? And if I do get out alive, what is it I am really supposed to be doing with my life?*

I had been asking myself similar questions ever since my first day at Antioch College, where I encountered just as many unanticipated challenges as I later faced on the volcanoes in Ecuador while serving in the Peace Corps.

Chapter 2

FIRST DAY OF COLLEGE

Yellow Springs, Ohio, September 1966

COMING FROM GERMANY, where I'd spent my last two years of high school, my first day at college back in the United States turned my world upside down.

My plane landed in Dayton, Ohio. As I walked from the jet bridge into the airport, I looked around with anticipation, having been notified that someone from the college would be holding a sign with my name on it.

When the crowd thinned, I finally saw a small, cardboard placard with the words "Erica Merriam" written in whimsical rainbow lettering. The guy holding it was tall and barefoot, with long, wildly disheveled hair and a curly beard. I glanced into his face; his shiny eyes looked back at me as though laughing. With fascination and a faint tinge of fear, I looked him over, trying to size up the situation.

I wonder if I'm safe riding with this strange character.

He reached out to shake my hand. As I stepped closer to him, an unfamiliar but pleasant scent, similar to burned leaves, wafted into my nose.

"Hey, man. What's happening. You Erica Merriam?"

"Yes, I am. Who are you?"

"I'm your ride. Let's get your bags and split. We gotta boogie to Yellow Springs so you can register before the office closes."

"What's your name?" I asked, trying to find some ground to stand on.

"Wolf Man."

"Wolf Man? What kind of name is that? American Indian? Is that your first or last name?"

"Just call me Wolf. That's good enough."

We bounced along in his bright orange spray-painted VW van on the long ride from Dayton to Yellow Springs. Through the window, cornfields stretched into the distance with their yellow harvested stalks, row after endless row. This was my first time in the Midwest, except for a few months I'd spent in Kansas as a newborn.

Wolf was friendly and talkative, which helped allay the mild discomfort from being in the hands of a stranger. Although he spoke English, many of the words and phrases he used were foreign to me. He asked if I had ever dropped acid.

"I don't remember having spilled any. Well, maybe once in chemistry class." He told me when he first took acid it blew his mind. I had no idea what he was talking about.

We drove into the leafy, green campus. It was a reassuring sight, with its historic brick buildings interspersed with modern classrooms and apartment complexes. In front of the student union, Wolf dropped me off with my luggage. "Keep your cool, baby," he said, flashing a peace sign. "See you around."

As I grabbed my bags, ready to walk up the stairs to register, I saw a cluster of disheveled people gathered off to one side of the building, intently watching something hidden from view. Curious, I put the bags down and walked over. In my stylish Florentine shoes with stacked heels, matching purse, and miniskirt, I stood next to the motley group of men and women and peered into the center until I saw the object of their attention. Air sucked into my chest as my hand went reflexively to cover my mouth. There was a naked man preaching to the group. I tapped the shoulder of the tall, long-haired young man standing next to me.

"Excuse me, sir. Can you please tell me what is happening here?"

"The dude's flipped out on acid," he said matter-of-factly.

"Oh, I see," I said, pretending I'd understood what he said.

> *Oh my God. This is a crazy place. I think I made a big mistake.*

I headed back to the student union to register for classes. The friendly, older woman who helped me with the paperwork spoke the same kind of English I did and wore a skirt and a blouse and had shoes on her feet, something I could identify with.

"Welcome to Yellow Springs, Ohio, and Antioch College," she said. "I'm Lynette Johnston. I imagine that Antioch will be an adjustment for you, coming from Germany. But we're here to help you in any way we can. Just come on in when you have any questions or problems, or you need someone to talk to over a cup of coffee."

> *What a relief that there is a normal person here. Maybe everything will be all right in the end, even if I just have one person I can talk to. How did I get so out of sync with American culture? I was only gone for two years.*

Mrs. Johnston interrupted my thoughts and asked if I had any more questions before I got settled in. Feeling a sense of kinship with her, I brought up the scene I'd just witnessed with the naked man.

"Mrs. Johnston, why don't the students here comb their hair? Why do some of them dress in rags—or walk around nearly naked?"

"Please, Erica, call me Lynette. We all call each other by our first names here."

Lynette explained that, unlike most colleges of that era, Antioch had no dress code, including no rules against being naked. She went on to say that Antioch was known to be progressively liberal, even radical. She confessed that she'd had a difficult time adjusting to Antioch when she first joined the staff, being from a conservative Midwestern family.

Lynette assured me that I would get a good education. She said that Antioch regularly turned out graduates who went on to become stellar public figures, such as civil rights activists Eleanor Holmes Norton and Coretta Scott King, wife of Martin Luther King, Jr.—and Rod Serling, creator of *The Twilight Zone*.

I'm in the Twilight Zone right here, right now.

Lynette said that I would eventually get used to this unusual college. She even predicted that I would come to love this place the way she had.

"I'm curious to know why you picked Antioch," she said, showing genuine interest.

During my junior year of high school, I had started thinking about which college would be right for me. In the office of the college counselor, I leafed through the thick catalog of US colleges. I looked at the pictures and read the information, but I couldn't get a sense of any of the schools. They all sounded the same. As an American student abroad, I'd received almost no guidance on how to choose a school. Many of my classmates simply chose colleges or universities that friends or relatives had attended. I was inclined to just do the same, until a twist of fate intervened the following summer.

In those days, hitchhiking offered a cheap and mostly safe means of getting around in Europe, even for girls. On a tight budget, I stayed in youth hostels during my summer travel adventures. At two different youth hostels in France, I had bumped into Antioch College students. They stood out from the other travelers with their colorful, gypsy-like garb, their guitars and harmonicas and free-spirited ways—juxtaposed with their worldly knowledge about politics and social issues. They seemed to have a fervent idealism and belief that they could change the world.

Listening to them talk was mesmerizing. But what really grabbed my attention was hearing that they were getting college credit for traveling and learning about other cultures. This convinced me that Antioch was the right choice.

That fall, I announced to my college counselor, Miss Brill, that I had made up my mind about where I intended to go to college. Upon hearing my choice, she frowned with disapproval and tried to persuade me to reconsider.

"Antioch is not a place for a nice, intelligent girl like you," she said emphatically.

"Why not?"

"There are liberals and radicals at that school. They go on marches and do a lot of protesting against our government. They're disruptive. And boys and girls are housed in the same dorm. Nothing good can come of that."

> *I've shared my living space with my two brothers my whole life. What's the problem?*

She added, "I've been told that the students smoke marijuana."

"What's that?" I asked.

"It's a plant that makes you do crazy and bad things." It sounded intriguing.

My parents read the catalogue about Antioch and learned that it was founded in 1852, based on egalitarian, liberal arts principles. It had admitted Black students during the time of slavery, and in the mid-1800s it became the first US school to appoint a woman as a full professor.

Antioch pioneered the work-study program called "co-operative education," shortened to "co-op," as part of its five-year curriculum. Half the year, students worked at their co-op jobs off campus in the "real" world, allowing them to combine their idealism on campus with down-to-earth practicality on the job.

Antioch had a reputation for producing socially engaged citizens. The college motto was a quote from Horace Mann, the college's first president: "Be ashamed to die until you have won some victory for humanity."

Based on what my parents read—and what I failed to disclose—they had no objections.

Lynette sat for a moment in silence with a smile on her face, as though digesting the story. She said she loved hearing about how students end up choosing Antioch.

I eagerly asked Lynette if Antioch offered a Junior Year Abroad program, like many of the Ivy League schools. She said they did not offer that specific program. She must have noticed the disappointed look on my face and asked me why this was important to me. I confessed to her that Jean Pierre, my French fiancé, and I had become engaged just before I left Europe. We planned to get married when I returned to Europe for my junior year abroad. I managed to hold back the tears.

Lynette asked one of the students who had wandered into the building to give me a quick orientation of the campus. The young woman, fittingly named "Sunny," cheerfully took on the role of tour guide. She was slender with bushy hair, some of which lay in rows of tiny braids in the front half of her head. Her *café au lait* skin emanated an attractive glow. She had on jeans that looked like the legs had been cut off—or torn off—to make them into shorts. There was no hem, just unanchored threads. When she bent over to pick an apple off the ground, I could see the edge of her butt. No underwear. She wore a T-shirt that revealed her nipples through the thin fabric. No bra. On her feet were leather sandals that looked handmade. Seeing me looking at them, she said, "Those are *huaraches*. I got them when I was down in Mexico, in San Miguel de Allende, studying Spanish."

As she led me around campus, Sunny told me she'd been offered generous scholarships at several top-notch schools. I asked her why she had chosen Antioch. She said that the students had a voice in how the school was governed. She loved the idea of the work-study program, and she was impressed by the college's history of being one of the first schools in the country to accept Black students and later to offer the co-op method of education. She said her ideas and politics were too radical for her to consider going to a conventional school. She was among kindred spirits at Antioch. "We're all eccentrics here, people who know how to think for themselves."

I wonder if I'm eccentric.

During my tour of the campus, Sunny took me to a place she went when she needed time alone to "process." Glen Helen Nature Preserve was a vast tract of land with forests, streams, and meadows. Wandering along a trail, we heard voices in the distance. Sunny said that the Peace Corps had been using the Preserve to train volunteers before they left for their assignments abroad.

We watched the volunteers do group bonding activities, including a ropes course strung between tall trees on opposite ends of a meadow where the participants helped each other get across to the other side. I could feel their excitement. I made a mental note to consider applying to the Peace Corps myself someday.

The tour ended at Birch Hall, the modern building that would be my dorm for the next year. After Sunny left, I found a pay phone and called my parents to let them know I had arrived safely. I described to them the beautiful campus, but I kept the conversation short, leaving out the aspects that troubled me.

Seeing that my dorm was empty, I went to my room, shut the door, and lay down on my narrow bed. I cried softly into the pillow, feeling lost and disoriented. I missed Jean Pierre terribly.

Did I make a mistake choosing Antioch College?

I had adjusted to several different cultures in my rather short lifetime. Surely I could adjust to college life in the 1960s. I decided the best place to begin was to adopt some of the customs of the host country—in this case, the host college.

Of course I ditched my miniskirts, heels, and purse the day after I arrived, exchanging them for jeans with handmade embroidery around the pockets, an embroidered blouse from Mexico, *huarache* sandals, and a cloth bag from Africa—all purchased from the secondhand store in the artsy-craftsy town of Yellow Springs. The store smelled like leaves burning on a fall day after raking. I had detected the same odor upon entering my dorm; it hung in the air like a cloud. As it turned out, this smell would become very familiar throughout my years in college.

Next on the agenda was learning the dialect and customs.

> *Maybe in the end, I'll fall in love with this place, like Lynette said. I just have to make sure my parents don't come for a visit while I'm here.*

Chapter 3

MY NEW LIFE

It wasn't long before the music of Bob Dylan, the Beatles, and the Rolling Stones woke me up to the unrest unfolding throughout the country. I memorized the stirring words to many of Dylan's songs and often sang them to myself.

The potpourri of sounds around campus included ethnic music that I found enchanting, like Ravi Shankar's trance-inducing sitar music, which wafted through the candlelit, incense-saturated dorms. Miriam Makeba, the South African singer and civil rights activist, stirred my heart to care about what was happening on another continent.

The passion for the music of those times served as part of the glue that held the students together. They had a common language that even I spoke.

Eventually the novelty of life on campus began to wear off, along with my feelings of isolation. I quickly learned the hip lingo of my classmates and adjusted to their freewheeling lifestyle. Budding friendships helped with the transition.

Antioch was a hotbed of political activism, avant-garde ideas, and social experimentation. I got a crash course in the US government's foreign policies, especially regarding the war in Vietnam. Politics came up in nearly every conversation.

When inquisitive friends asked about my parents, I didn't dare mention that my father had been a general in the US Army—even though he didn't agree with our country's actions in Vietnam. Instead, I spoke about his new career as dean of students at a college in New Hampshire and his love of academia.

Despite all the marches and demonstrations happening around me, politics did not hold the highest place on my life agenda. A compelling need for self-discovery consumed most of my energy as I attempted to sort out where and how I fit into this new world.

Academic life at Antioch had little structure and hardly resembled what I had expected from college. The college had abolished letter and number grades in favor of individualized written evaluations by the professors, in an attempt to elevate students' love of learning above our desire to get good grades. Coming from an intensely competitive background, I felt disoriented by this concept.

Freshmen took multiple tests shortly after arriving on campus so that the faculty could get an idea of our academic strengths and weaknesses. If we scored high enough, the basic requirements would be waived. I tested out of several classes, including all math and science, thanks to the rigorous education I had received in Germany.

This taste of freedom was exciting—and scary. Incredulous at the thought of no grades and no required science classes, I wondered whether I would accomplish anything in college. But I soon got over the feelings of guilt at wasting my parents' money on tuition and jumped at the opportunity to sign up for all the fun courses I could find that first semester, like stained-glass window making, pottery, piano, theater, and geology. In the early mornings, I joined a dedicated group of students for yoga and meditation. I also joined an informal discussion group that focused on popular books and their relevance to the times, including *Zen and the Art of Motorcycle Maintenance,* and the importance of being fully engaged in life.

Theater was a class that I looked forward to each week. The director gave me several roles in little sketches by Harold Pinter, Samuel Beckett, and several off-Broadway playwrights. He told me I should consider a career in acting. I loved to act and poured my heart into it. I took a special interest in trying to get inside the characters I played, imagining that I was seeing the world through their eyes. This trait served me well in developing empathy for others who were different from me.

The living situation at Antioch defied accepted standards of that era. There were, indeed, men in the dorm building—just as Miss Brill had warned. In fact, Antioch was one of the first schools in the nation to have co-ed dorms. But being in such close quarters with men had the opposite effect on me from what my counselor had worried about. The mystery of "otherness" that fuels romantic sparks dissipated rapidly with the routine familiarity of the opposite sex. The men left the toilet seats up in the bathroom and made messes. It wasn't that different from living with my brothers.

The dorms had no adult supervision. Casual sex, drugs, and loud music were pervasive. Peer pressure to join in on the fun was strong. I managed to evade the casual sex, but my irrepressible curiosity led me through a short-lived phase of indulging in everything the school had to offer, including cigarettes, alcohol, junk food, candy, sodas, pot, psychedelic mushrooms, and LSD. In short order, I became emotionally unstable, exacerbated by sleep deprivation.

I experienced an ongoing state of minor psychosis, marked by distorted thoughts and by what was then called manic depression with huge swings of mood and energy. No one seemed to notice.

After a few months, the thrill of engaging in these illicit activities wore off. I lost interest in the drugs and alcohol. This route did not appear to be my path and made me feel like my life had no purpose.

My roommate, Loretta, came from Wyoming, a place in the Wild West beyond my limited mental map. The unrefined, free, and easy way about her struck me as both foreign and fascinating. I envied the way she moved through her day with what appeared to be relaxed and unquestioning confidence, free of the angst and doubt that I thought were an everyday aspect of the human condition. Loretta's mantra was "Don't worry. Everything will be fine."

> *How is it possible not to worry? Maybe in the West they don't understand that there's a lot to worry about in the world.*

The dorm room was small. Our beds stood at right angles to each other. Several nights a week, Loretta's newly acquired boyfriend spent the night in her narrow bed. The squeaking bed springs, the grunting and moaning sounds of sex at close range, and the sharp smell of bodily fluids rattled my mind and robbed me of my sleep. I didn't dare protest, knowing they'd think I was uncool and prudish.

In geology class, a student caught my eye one day when he looked at me across the aisle. He had a slender body with blond hair, pale skin, and piercing blue eyes. He resembled a contemporary version of Adonis with a black leather jacket and matching black pants. He stared at me long and hard in class with his electric blue eyes, in a way that I couldn't ignore. Overcome with shyness and awkwardness, I had to look away. My face flushed and my heart raced. Good thing there were no grades at Antioch, because I could no longer pay attention to what the professor was saying.

At the end of class, I dashed off, too shy to make contact with the handsome student. But before leaving, I leaned over and asked the woman next to me for his name. She answered, "Jeff Elliott."

I enjoyed the attention I received from other male students as well. Jim from Kentucky, with his melodious voice and soft Southern accent, took a shine to me and invited me to spend the weekend with him at his family's cattle and tobacco farm. He would become a lifelong loyal friend.

Anonymous notes, each with the same handwriting, came every few days to my student mailbox—love notes with little colored ink drawings and quotes from *Le Petit Prince* and other sources. It was exciting not knowing who the author of the notes was. Every man I knew who might be a possibility denied having written the beautiful notes. The author never revealed himself.

While adapting to life at college, I tried at the same time to remain faithful to Jean Pierre in Paris, my first love from high school days, and whose family-heirloom engagement ring I wore on my finger.

Chapter 4

MARRIAGE

MAINTAINING A FANTASY-LIKE RELATIONSHIP with Jean Pierre in France added to my existential disorientation while coping with the foreign and often bizarre world of Antioch. I felt like I was leading a split life.

In spite of our oaths to be faithful to each other forever and ever, and in spite of my promise to spend my junior year abroad at the Sorbonne in Paris, where we would get married, I began thinking less and less of Jean Pierre. I eventually stopped writing him letters and took off his engagement ring. The sweet and tender memories of our summer together seemed to belong to someone else. I was undergoing some very drastic changes.

In second-semester geology, I spotted Jeff Elliott once again in my class. After a few days of his disarming stares across the aisle, he introduced himself and asked if I wanted to go for a ride on his motorcycle. We drove all over Yellow Springs on Jeff's Triumph. I sat behind him with my arms encircling his waist. I noticed how exciting it felt to be touching his body.

Jeff lived off campus, having earned that privilege by virtue of being a sophomore. There was an air of mystery about him. He spoke cryptically, injecting quotes from Bob Dylan songs into his speech. "Oh, Mama. Can this really be the end, to be stuck inside of Mobile with the Memphis blues again?"

His mind worked in mysterious ways. I discovered that he had used hallucinogens heavily in his first year of college and had experienced disturbing flashbacks from his LSD trips.

When I told Jeff about my difficulty sleeping during my roommate's nocturnal sexual activities, he invited me to live with him in his apartment off campus. After that, we became truly inseparable. We walked everywhere arm in arm, hand in hand. When one of my college friends saw us together, she commented that we looked like two children lost in the woods.

We fell madly in love. I had never experienced so much attention and adoration. Life on a pedestal felt irresistible. I had no idea at the time that a pedestal is a precarious place to be because there's only one way to go after being perched so high, and that's down.

Jeff took me to Illinois to meet his parents, Edith and Oz, who welcomed me into their family with warmth and enthusiasm. A few months later, as we were walking hand in hand in the Glen Helen Nature Preserve, we stopped near a small waterfall. Jeff turned to me and reached out to hold both of my hands. He looked straight into my eyes and said, "Erica, I adore you. I'm crazy about you. I want you to be with me for the rest of my life. Will you marry me?"

I knew that I had become addicted to Jeff's intoxicating attention and fervent expressions of love and admiration. I didn't want them to end. In my naïve young mind, marriage appeared to be a way to secure that devotion. I said, "Yes."

My parents approved of Jeff. He came from a family of means and he treated me well. Back in that era, parents felt good about marrying off their daughters before they became "old maids."

On December 27, 1967, I became Jeff's wife. I was nineteen.

With my marriage to Jeff, I gave up my family name, Merriam, and switched to Elliott. I practiced saying my new name over and over. "My name is Erica Elliott." I liked the way it sounded. The new name symbolized a new life and gave me some psychological distance from my family. I wanted to free myself from their expectations and judgments as I struggled to find my own way in the world as an adult.

Jeff's parents owned an elegant home in an upscale neighborhood south of Chicago. While visiting, I saw several stunning black-and-white photographs hanging on the walls throughout their mansion. When I inquired about them, I learned that Jeff had taken the photographs. His mother said her son was extremely artistic, especially in the area of photography.

Oz was president of a thriving local bank, and Jeff could have whatever material possessions he wanted. The family shared what they had with Jeff and me at every opportunity. Oz even insisted on paying for my college tuition after we were married, even though my parents certainly had the means to pay for my tuition themselves. Such exceptional generosity left me feeling disoriented.

My Swiss mother had raised her six children in her culture's tradition of frugality. Even though my mother came from a well-off doctor's family and my father was a high-ranking officer, my mother taught us not to waste anything, to eat everything on our plates, and to save practically everything–even things we didn't need. She made soup out of table scraps, she recycled the dishwater on the houseplants, and she used paper and strings over and over until they disintegrated. We wore hand-me-down clothes that Mummy patched and darned so artfully that we still looked presentable and lived up to her high standards of propriety and cleanliness.

My three sisters and I learned how to sew because, if we wanted some special piece of clothing, we had to make it ourselves. When I was in the tenth grade, my sisters and I sewed our own fashionable silk brocade A-line dresses for the memorable opening of the Bolshoi Ballet in Washington, DC.

As college kids, Jeff and I owned a brand-new Ford Mustang convertible, and we each had our own motorcycle; mine was a Kawasaki. During school breaks, Edith and Oz took us to a resort in Mexico, where we lounged on the beach and sipped margaritas, and to a dude ranch in Colorado, where we rode horses in the mountains.

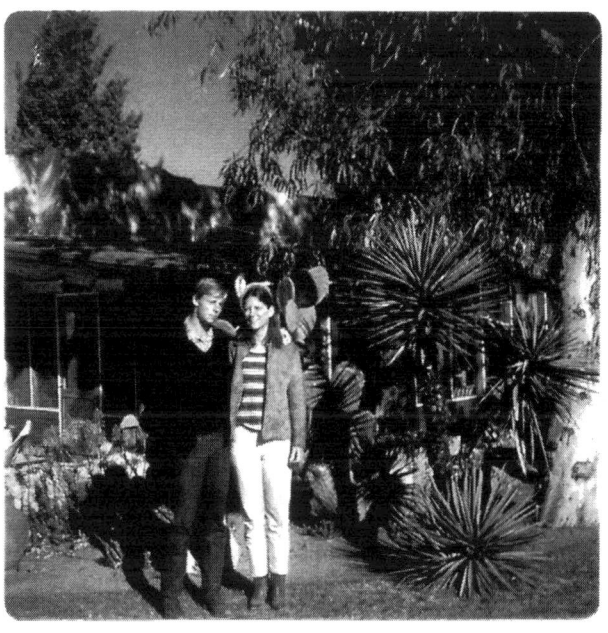

Jeff and me on spring break in Tucson, Arizona, 1968

By today's standards, what we had would not be considered exceptional for a college kid, but in those days it was like living in a fantasy world. In fact, at times I felt embarrassed to be living in such luxury while my classmates struggled to make ends meet. Many students came from wealthy families but chose a life of poverty—or pretended they were poor. It wasn't cool in the 1960s to be rich or too interested in money, at least not at Antioch.

Having anything I wanted in the material realm had an exhilarating effect initially, but the thrill wore off over time. I began to miss the feelings of excitement and appreciation for small things, and the sense of accomplishment that comes from working hard for what one has. Paradoxically, this new material wealth made me feel impoverished in my inner world. It contributed to my growing feelings that my current life had no purpose.

Being married while we were students was an anomaly at Antioch, like practicing a custom from a different era. While I made a dedicated effort to suppress my wild spirit and mold myself into a "good" wife according to some outdated cultural script, the sexual revolution was happening all around me. It was a time of free love, the birth control pill, and women's liberation. I felt out of sync with the times, just as I had so often since coming to Antioch.

As part of Antioch's work-study program, Jeff and I landed co-op jobs that spring in Cambridge, Massachusetts, where my sister Vreni lived while attending Harvard for graduate studies in Chinese. Jeff studied photography with his mentor, Minor White, while I worked at a well-known mental hospital just outside of Boston. During the previous quarter on campus, I had taken a course in psychology and had developed an intense interest in this field—probably in an attempt to understand the workings of my inner self. I wanted to translate what I had learned in the classroom into hands-on experiential learning.

My job as a psychiatric nursing assistant required me to spend time with patients and report back to the nurses my findings from the day, a kind of tattling clothed in the guise of treatment.

Instead of merely gathering data, as though I were studying strange animal behavior in a zoo, I developed friendships with the patients. They didn't seem that different from me, except that most of them were overtly unhappy, sometimes moaning and crying.

"I'm not crazy! I don't belong here!" one woman yelled. "Get me out of here. Someone help me get out of here. I want to go home!" She had confessed to me earlier that she had spit out her Thorazine because the medication left her feeling like a zombie.

Over time, I became fond of the patients. I brought them little snacks and other treats, listened intently to their stories, rubbed their feet while they lay in bed, and naïvely appointed myself as their advocate, speaking to the staff on their behalf in order to improve conditions.

To my surprise, the staff did not appreciate my self-appointed role as patient advocate. Around a month into the job, the supervisor summoned me to his office.

"Your advocacy for the patients suggests an over-identification with them," he said. "To help you with this over-identification problem, I recommend that you see a therapist." When I declined the offer to see a therapist and tried to justify my actions, he said it would probably be best if I resigned. I asked what would happen if I didn't resign. "You will be fired," he said matter-of-factly.

A few minutes later, in a daze of disbelief, I gathered my things from my locker and left the big brick building for the last time, without saying goodbye to the patients. I could barely breathe from the crushing feelings of shame and bewilderment.

When I tearfully told Jeff that I had been fired, he burst into laughter. Comforting me, he said that being fired from "Mt. Misery Mental Hospital" was something to be proud of. Nonetheless, I made him swear never to tell anyone, especially not our parents.

Back on campus, turmoil and upheaval reigned. It was 1968. NASA had just launched the Apollo 7 spacecraft to the moon. Anti-war demonstrations had reached a high pitch. Being married and living off campus, I found myself looking on as a bystander, trying to make sense out of the explosive times we were living in.

Jeff and I spent one of our three-month co-op jobs together in San Francisco. I did clerical work in a bank where Jeff's father had found me a position, while Jeff studied art and photography at the San Francisco Art Institute.

Even though the women's liberation movement had begun, I was still stuck in a bygone era. I tried hard to please Jeff and support his future in photography, even if it meant overlooking my own needs. If I were single, I would never have considered working in a bank. Clerical work had no appeal to me.

It was a heady time in San Francisco. The anti-war demonstrations and the antics of the hippies of Haight-Ashbury dominated the news, along with the discussions about the use of pot and hallucinogens. My little world orbited on the periphery of the psychedelic part of San Francisco. I looked on in fascination, like a tourist in a foreign culture.

A year after our time in San Francisco, we spent a semester in San Miguel de Allende, Mexico. We lived in a beautiful villa we had rented, complete with spacious grounds and a woman who cooked and cleaned for us. I felt more like a traveler on a prolonged five-star vacation than a student in college during such tumultuous times.

In San Miguel, Jeff continued his studies in photography, while I studied Spanish, weaving, and silver jewelry making at the Instituto Allende. Every day we shopped at the outdoor food market, and every few days we explored the surrounding countryside. In those days, San Miguel was a quaint and colorful little village, just beginning to attract a stream of expats from the States.

While on some level I was thoroughly enjoying the luxury that came from living with Jeff, there were uncomfortable rumblings deep within me, portending that something was very wrong. Doubts began percolating to the surface about the path I was on. I had an increasingly pervasive feeling that I had lost my way and that I was aimlessly drifting through my college years without any real purpose.

I sensed that my life did indeed have a distinct purpose, but I had no idea what that purpose was. I wondered how I could find the key that would reveal the information I needed. The complete freedom and lack of structure in college had left me feeling lost, without a map and compass, without a guide. I felt as if I had stepped into someone else's life, cast in a role that I wasn't suited for. I was confused and unable to articulate those vague feelings of discontent in the midst of a seemingly enviable lifestyle.

I fell into a state of despair and angst that I now understand in retrospect was serious existential depression.

Chapter 5

BREAKDOWN

Once Jeff and I returned to the Antioch campus to resume our studies, I began to unravel. Life seemed simply meaningless. The chaos and disintegration of old ways in the culture around me mirrored the chaos and disintegration of the person I used to be. I became aimless and despondent. I disliked myself and projected my feelings onto Jeff. We began to argue and say and do hurtful things to each other. My unrealistic fantasies of how a marriage was supposed to be crumbled. I blamed myself for the arguments and concluded that I was a bad person.

In psychology class I learned about anorexia and bulimia and how some people, especially girls and women, use food to cope with anxiety and depression, low self-esteem, and a distorted self-image. In an attempt to gain some control over my life and my feelings, I became anorexic for a few weeks and then bulimic. I lost a lot of weight, thinking that being skinny would make Jeff love me more. The induced vomiting did not purge my feelings of worthlessness, though, so I dropped the anorexia and bulimia and tried other approaches.

During this time of inner turbulence and despair, my older sister Jackie, with whom I'd been close as a young girl, and her husband Alan, both college professors, had been awarded fellowships to teach for a year, by coincidence, at Antioch as visiting scholars.

While they were at Antioch, I made almost no contact with them, even though they were important people in my life.

On my spiral downward into depression, I tried to separate myself from my family. I could no longer play the old roles, and yet I hadn't found a new role for myself. I didn't want my sister to see me in this state of disintegration. The structure of my old self had collapsed and there was nothing yet to take its place.

Jeff saw how unhappy I was and assumed he was the problem. He swung back and forth between giving me an extra dose of love to giving me exasperation-fueled advice about how to fix myself. Usually, these discussions ended in arguments and tears.

One day, as I sailed down a hill on my bicycle in the countryside a few miles outside of Yellow Springs, pedaling as fast as I could to release pent-up emotions, I hit a patch of gravel and swerved off the road. My body tumbled over an embankment and down into a gulch, landing among the lower branches of a sycamore tree. My chest was so painful I could barely breathe. A man who saw the accident painstakingly extracted me from the tree and took me to the hospital. The ER doctor patched up my scrapes, x-rayed my cracked ribs, and put me in a brace. I declined the pain medication. The outer pain served as a distraction from my inner pain and torment.

After the bicycle accident, I could no longer avoid facing how unhappy I was with my life and with myself. While lost in my ruminations, I got the idea that it would be better if I were not around anymore. Having read French and German literature of the Romantic era in which suicide was considered noble, usually related to unrequited love, I considered this possibility for myself— although in my case, suicide would be for an unrequited search for my soul.

On a dreary and overcast day, while Jeff was in class on campus, I went into the kitchen in our apartment, opened the white oven door, pulled up a chair next to the open oven, and then turned on the gas, recreating what I had read in the literature. I waited. Nothing happened. I couldn't smell any gas. Assuming the pilot light had gone out, I leaned over to get a closer look into the oven and struck a match. The instant the match lit, an explosion shook the building and blasted me backwards, still in my wooden chair, smashing me against the back wall of the tiny kitchen.

A burnt smell filled my nose and sinuses. I could feel that the explosion had singed my eyebrows and the hair above my forehead. Our second-floor neighbor heard the explosion and rushed into our apartment. He grabbed me, threw me into the cold shower to put out the smoldering fire in my hair, then ran back into the kitchen and threw water on areas that were still burning. Miraculously, no major damage was done—except that my attempt had failed and I was still alive.

What now?

The neighbor sensed that this was not an accident and told the dean of students what had happened. The dean called me into her office. She was a kind, matronly woman, well known to me, whom I held in high regard. During this encounter, her voice sounded stern. She said she had no alternative but to notify my parents. I begged her not to tell them what had happened. I said I would do anything she wanted me to do if she would just not tell them. She said I would have to see the local psychiatrist and have regular sessions with him.

When I looked hesitant, the dean said that if I didn't agree to see the psychiatrist, she would have to tell my parents and I would be dismissed from college. I reluctantly agreed. The dean picked up the phone and made an appointment for me for the very next day, not giving me much time to back out.

The following day I rode my motorcycle to downtown Yellow Springs and found the nineteenth-century red brick office building where the psychiatrist worked. I took a deep breath, heaved open the glass door, and walked in, barely breathing. A woman in a red dress with vintage jeweled cat eyeglasses sat behind a desk smoking a cigarette. She smiled at me with a look of pity and handed me a form to fill out. Fortunately, she didn't ask me why I was there. Her potent patchouli perfume helped disguise the strong smell of cigarette smoke that filled the waiting room. Soft rock music of the elevator genre played in the background. Ashtrays scattered on little tables throughout the room were full to the brim. Obviously lots of nervous people had waited here.

After I had squirmed in my seat and chewed on my nails for about half an hour, a Black man in a tailored suit walked into the waiting room with hand extended. "Hello. My name is Dr. Samuels. I assume you are Erica Elliott." He stood tall, with good posture, like he was proud of himself—in contrast to my contracted state. We shook hands. I tried to look him in the eyes, but I was overcome with shame and merely looked fleetingly in the direction of his face, long enough to see that Dr. Samuels was handsome with dark brown skin, high cheekbones, and intense greenish-brown eyes.

In his office, Dr. Samuels sat down in his big swivel chair behind a large, cherry wood desk and puffed on his pipe. His desk had several piles of paper and a few framed pictures of children. There were prints on the wall by Picasso, Chagall, and Cezanne, and a few other artists I didn't recognize. In one corner, several large potted plants added some life to the serious atmosphere. Soothing sounds of running water in a fountain came from somewhere in the room.

Dr. Samuels motioned me to sit in the chair in front of his desk. I felt mortally ashamed, embarrassed to be in the room with a psychiatrist, especially a handsome one. In those days, therapy was reserved mostly for people in mental hospitals with serious conditions, like paranoid schizophrenia and psychosis—similar to the patients I looked after at Mt. Misery Mental Hospital outside of Boston.

Our session began by Dr. Samuels listing his outstanding credentials, including his degree in psychiatry from Zurich, Switzerland. From there he launched into our first counseling session. He said that I had made a "suicide gesture," which was essentially a call for help.

He spoke in a deep, clear voice with no discernible accent from any specific geographical area. After talking a bit in generalities, he began asking me highly personal questions about myself. I looked at the floor and cried quietly, without speaking. My stomach felt tight and my breathing restricted. Dr. Samuels handed me a box of Kleenex and kept asking questions. I remained silent, too mortified to speak.

The hour passed. He gave me a slip of paper with the time and date of our next appointment. I managed to mumble, "Thank you," while still looking at the floor. It was a relief to get out of there.

The following week I returned to Dr. Samuels' office with dread. We began the session the same way as before. He asked questions and I responded with silence, eyes glued to the floor. After a long pause, Dr. Samuels said, crisply enunciating each word, "I want you to leave now. You do not need to return. We are done." He walked to the door and held it open.

I looked up at him with utter surprise. "You don't want me to come back?" I said, incredulous.

"No. Don't come back."

I pleaded, "But I have to come back or else the dean will tell my parents about what happened, and I'll be asked to leave Antioch."

"You can come back when you're ready to talk and participate in your treatment."

"Okay, I'll talk."

Chapter 6

ARCHEOLOGY OF THE SOUL

Dr. Samuels won my trust and gently coaxed me into talking about my life. Once I started talking, I couldn't stop.

The therapy sessions became a sanctuary for me, a place where I could safely reveal my deepest truths without shame. He listened with uninterrupted and disarming empathy. My finely tuned radar did not detect even a trace of ridicule or judgment—something I had never experienced before, at least not in my family.

I felt deeply seen and heard for the first time in my life, which in itself had a significantly therapeutic effect—even without Dr. Samuels giving me any advice.

Holding this space enabled me to safely sort out my problems and gain insights into the childhood origins of some of my dysfunctional behavior and the emotional pain that tormented me.

I saw Dr. Samuels every week that I was on campus during my last two years of college, sometimes even twice a week. Jeff's father generously paid for the therapy. The sessions became an adventure that I looked forward to immensely.

Working with Dr. Samuels felt like studying the archeology of the soul. It involved a lot of digging, putting pieces together, exposing harmful myths and misperceptions, and looking at the past with a new perspective.

After each session, I returned to our apartment off campus and wrote down in a spiral-bound notebook the gist of what Dr. Samuels had said, along with some of the insights I'd learned through talking with him.

As we shed light on the forces that shaped my life, the first glimmer of compassion for myself bubbled to the surface.

At first, Dr. Samuels focused on my dreams. Having studied psychiatry in Zurich, he must have been influenced by Carl Jung's work in dream interpretation.

In one of my recurring dreams, I'm walking through a big city when I suddenly become aware that I have no clothes on. I feel mortified and ashamed. These dreams had plagued me when I was a teenager and my body was going through rapid changes. Dr. Samuels suggested that the dreams might also come from a fear of being my truest self.

Then there were the dreams of being stuck inside an elevator, in a state of panic, with no way to escape the endless ride up and down. These may have been about my inability to escape from a pre-scripted life into a more authentic one, in alignment with my soul's longings.

Another recurring dream appeared soon after Jeff and I got married. I'm the captain of a ship out at sea. Everything seems to be going smoothly until I realize I have no compass. I have no idea where we are or where we're headed. When the crew finds out that I don't know where we're going, they rebel and want to throw me overboard. At that moment, a storm brews, the water churns with turbulence, and the ship is on the verge of capsizing when I wake up out of breath.

Some of my dreams in high school, verging on nightmares, had a consistent theme about being lost and afraid in the face of great danger. In one, I'm a Jewish woman in a perpetual state of breathless flight from the Nazis who are bearing down on me. The dream first occurred in Germany after my father took my brother and me to visit Dachau, the concentration camp where thousands of Jews were murdered in the gas chambers. In the dream I'm naked. My head is shaved. I'm running for my life between row after row of barracks, with fierce barking dogs biting at my heels. I turn and look. Behind the dogs, the same SS guards who shaved my head are chasing me. I know they want to catch me and throw me into the gas chamber. I'm running as fast as I can, but they keep gaining on me. I glance behind again as one of the guards raises his pistol, about to strike me. I gasp for air—and find myself sitting upright in my bed, in the midst of a silent scream.

"Why do you think you dreamed about being a persecuted Jewish woman?" Dr. Samuels asked.

I told Dr. Samuels about the time I skipped school and took the trolley to the courthouse in downtown Frankfurt, where I attended a trial of some of the Auschwitz criminals who had surfaced long after the Nuremberg trials. It was the first time the German government put on trial its own wartime criminals.

The only seat available was in the Jewish section. During the trial it was hard for me to understand all of the legal talk at the front of the large courtroom, but I could see how angry the people were who sat near me. The woman right next to me quietly cried during the entire proceedings. A sense of alliance with the Jewish people welled up inside me. Although I kept silent, I wanted to say to the woman next to me, *Ich bin Jude in meinem Herzen*, "I am a Jew in my heart. I am with you."

Both experiences—visiting the death camp and witnessing the trials—seriously impacted my 16-year-old psyche and left me not only with recurrent nightmares, but also with disturbing existential questions.

> *How was it possible that those ordinary-looking men on trial had turned into such monsters, capable of pure cruelty and sadism? How did an entire nation get so completely indoctrinated that they turned against their Jewish neighbors? For the people with a conscience, were the personal risks of doing what was right too great during that time of darkness and deception?*

I wondered what it takes to make a good person turn into a bad person.

Dr. Samuels asked, "Are you wondering if you are capable of doing bad things, given the right circumstances?"

"Yes, I was wondering about that. I think I'd rather die than harm someone under any circumstances. But I guess we can't really know that for sure. I remember a time when my father did something bad because of certain circumstances."

"It's time we talked about your relationship with your father," Dr. Samuels said.

Chapter 7

MY FATHER AND ME

Eventually Dr. Samuels left the dream exploration behind and asked me many probing questions about my childhood. He questioned me specifically about my relationship with my father. He said he'd like to hear about the role my father played in my life.

My father and I had been buddies since I was a little girl. He already had three daughters and one son by the time I came along, so I suspect he might have been hoping for another son. My older brother, George, never formed a solid bond with my father. George was born while my father was away fighting in World War II. During that time, George developed a strong attachment to my mother and viewed my father as an intruder when he returned home at the end of the war.

I sensed my father's desire to do activities with a son and unconsciously accommodated his wish by becoming a tomboy. Even my childhood nickname, Rickie, sounded boyish—a shortened version of Erica, a name I shared with my mother.

Growing up, I adored my father. I wanted to be like him. He was a highly decorated war hero who still led an adventurous life—and, best of all, he was kind. I sensed he enjoyed being with me, especially in the outdoors.

My father was often gone on various assignments for the military and spent little time at home—like most fathers during that era. When he was home, I performed amazing feats to get his attention, knowing I had to compete with five attention-starved siblings. I even dove off the high diving board when I was only seven—just to win my father's approval.

My father stood at the edge of the pool, beer in hand, conversing with a group of men. "Daddy, look at me!" I called out. "Watch me dive off. Daddy, are you watching?" He looked up at me and smiled.

I was terrified being up so high with the water far below, but the prize would be worth it. Standing at the very edge of the board with trembling legs, I took a deep breath and dove off. As I sailed through the air, I looked over to make sure my father was watching.

He's not watching. He's talking with his friends.

I lost focus and did a belly flop, which knocked the wind out of me. The lifeguard helped pull me out of the water. My father walked over to comfort me as I stood at the edge of the pool, doubled over in pain. I had learned to be a good soldier and didn't complain. I resolved to find some other way to get his approval.

My father took me hiking, taught me basic rock-climbing skills, and even taught me how to shoot a pistol and a rifle at a shooting range. Although I did not have the least bit of interest in guns, at my father's suggestion I became a member of the local junior gun club, whose members were almost exclusively boys. During that year, I received two awards for good marksmanship. My father, obviously pleased, said, "Rickie, I'm proud of you." His comment meant the world to me.

My mother appeared chronically overwhelmed and exhausted by her rambunctious children. My parents decided to send the youngest children off to camp all summer, giving my mother a three-month reprieve. I got sent to a camp in Maine for six summers in a row.

At camp I learned many exciting skills, including horseback riding, canoeing, archery, water skiing, and competitive swimming. I also learned survival skills, like how to use an axe to chop down trees and brush for shelters, find my way in the wilderness using a map and compass, survive on roots and berries, and administer basic first aid.

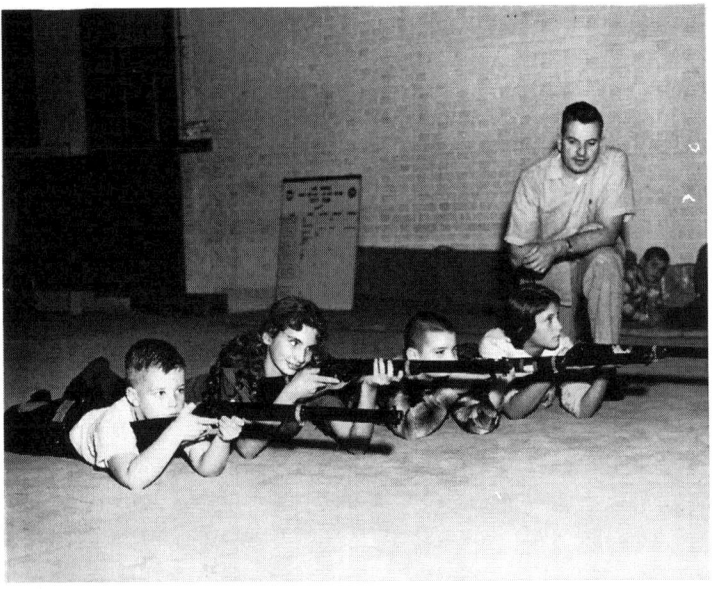

You'll find me on the far right, age ten, the only girl in the Rifle and Gun Club. I had no interest in guns, but I agreed to join the club to please my father during my tomboy phase.

With the skills I learned at camp, along with added training in wilderness survival, I qualified for the coveted Junior Maine Guide certification. The camp sent me to the governor's mansion in Augusta to receive my award and attend a ceremony in honor of the handful of young guides—mostly boys. I could feel my father's approval by the way he smiled and put his arm around me, like I was his buddy.

My father's approval was my life raft, an antidote to the crippling criticism and harsh judgments that prevailed in my family, especially from my mother.

When I was ten, we lived near the Chesapeake Bay in Ft. Monroe, Virginia. One weekend my father took me in his cabin cruiser down the Dismal Swamp Canal, just the two of us. It was thrilling to know that we were cruising a route used by the Underground Railroad, where escaped slaves traveled on their way to freedom in the North. Some of them had stayed and settled on the tiny islands in the swamp. But what was even more exciting to me than the local history was the chance to spend exclusive time with my father and not have to compete with anyone for his attention. I felt immensely lucky.

My mother used hitting, slapping, and spanking to gain some measure of control over her daughters. My two brothers were mostly spared from this kind of punishment. My mother seemed to favor the boys. I received more than my share of the physical punishment because I talked back and rebelled. Around the time I turned 11 years old, I noticed that I was taller than my mother. This gave me the nerve to defend myself.

As was common in those days, Mummy was angry with me for something I had done. When she raised her arm to hit me, I reached up and grabbed it in midair, and growled fiercely between clenched teeth, "Don't you dare hit me ever again." My mother looked shaken.

When my father came home from work that evening, Mummy told him I needed a "good spanking." Following my mother's orders, my father led me into a room at the back of the house. I had the strong impression that he did not enjoy spanking me and only did it at my mother's request. He closed the door as I braced myself for the familiar pain. What happened next took me by surprise and changed my life.

My father put one hand against my bottom, palm up, and clapped his hands together, making a loud noise. He told me to yell out as if in pain. I yelled. Then he sat down and spoke in a serious tone of voice.

"Rickie, you've got to try your best to cooperate with your mother and stop talking back to her. She has her hands full taking care of all of you children. I don't want to have to spank you anymore when I come home in the evening."

"I can't help it, Daddy. Mummy can be really mean. I don't like it when she keeps hitting me. She even hits me around my head when I play the wrong notes during piano practice. She thinks I do it on purpose to make her mad."

My father looked straight into my eyes and said, "Rickie, listen to me. I believe in you. I know that someday you're going to do something with your life that will make us very proud of you. You have a lot of spunk. You can do anything you put your mind to. Just try to cooperate right now with your mother, all right?"

I listened intently to what he had to say, taking his words literally.

> *He believes in me. He thinks I can do anything I put my mind to.*

My father's words had a mesmerizing effect on me. They made their way deep inside my soul and lodged there permanently, providing a talisman I would hold onto through times of self-doubt and feelings of worthlessness.

Dr. Samuels asked, "Did the hitting and spankings continue?"

"That incident marked the last attempt my mother ever made to hit me. I never got spanked again either."

My father said something else that helped me get through some very rough times later in life. When I turned 15, I was old enough in the state of Virginia to get my driver's license. What a thrill it was to drive the little blue Fiat my father had bought for his children to share. One afternoon I drove from my home in Arlington across the bridge to Washington, DC, where I took classes in sculpture at the Corcoran Art Gallery. On the way back, I had to suddenly slam on the brakes to avoid hitting a pedestrian in the street, causing the car behind to rear-end me and put a big dent into the little Fiat.

I was terrified to tell my father. I hated to disappoint him. Getting up all my nerve, I asked him if I could speak to him in private. In tears, I confessed to the accident and admitted that it was my fault. I waited for the guillotine to fall. Instead, after a brief silence, my father said in a kind voice, "Rickie, I'm glad this little accident happened to you. You learned an important lesson that fortunately did not cause you any injury. Now you will become an excellent driver."

I stood speechless, trying to digest his unexpected words of kindness and support. I did indeed become an excellent driver with a near-spotless record—except for parking tickets. Of even more significance, I learned that I could turn misfortune into something that could benefit me in the long run—an important life lesson.

Chapter 8

AT THE PUB

"W᯽ haven't talked much about your parents' relationship during your childhood. How did your parents meet and what attracted them to each other?" Dr. Samuels inquired.

My parents met in Switzerland. As a young man fresh out of Harvard grad school, my father taught science to high school students. To make extra money on the side, he tutored students at the Massachusetts Institute of Technology (MIT) in math. After two years of teaching, my father joined a teacher exchange program that placed him in England. Soon after arriving, my father befriended a fellow exchange student from Switzerland. His Swiss colleague, Heinz, invited him to travel with him back home for the Christmas holidays. While there, Heinz introduced my father to a beautiful woman, Erica Bauer, who was the goddaughter of his parents. My father instantly fell for her, struck by her beauty, her fine features, her soft accent, and her charming personality.

After my father returned to England, he and my mother exchanged heated love letters. At the end of the school year, my father returned to Switzerland to marry my mother. They married on the Matterhorn. Everyone in the wedding party wore hiking boots, including the priest, as they hiked up the steep slope to the tiny chapel.

Dr. Samuels asked, "Did the happiness last?"

At the Pub

Their happiness in the marriage lasted a few years. Soon after their wedding, they sailed on an ocean liner back to America and set up house together. My father resumed teaching science and math.

My two older sisters were toddlers and my brother George was on the way when my father left to fight in World War II. My mother had a rough time living with her mother-in-law, who pressured her to do things "the American way," like bottle-feeding her babies. Tensions were high as my mother resisted the pressure.

When my father returned from the war, it was as though my mother and father had become strangers. They had difficulty getting along. My mother was exhausted from having been a single mother during the war years. She became highly critical and resentful of my father and suspected him of having an affair during the war.

The post-war years, with my father gone much of the time due to his military duties, were tough for my mother. She appeared to be constantly overwhelmed looking after her six children.

"Did your father remain faithful to your mother?" Dr. Samuels asked.

My father cheated on my mother, which broke my heart and caused me to change my view of him. The consequences of my outrage at his betrayal of our family surprisingly led to a deeper understanding of life and feelings of compassion for both of my parents.

"Can you explain what you mean by that?" Dr. Samuels asked.

In 1961, around the time I entered my early teens, my father left for an assignment in Korea as secretary of the United Nations peacekeeping mission at Panmunjom in the demilitarized zone between North and South Korea. The army called service in Asia (then referred to as "the Orient") "hardship tours" because officers went alone without their families.

After my father left for his hardship tour, all hell broke loose in the family. My mother coped as best she could while we kids ran wild—fighting with each other, staying out late, and getting into trouble. I missed my father and his guiding influence on me. Without his natural air of authority to keep at least a semblance of peace, my mother was in a persistent state of agitation and exasperation. She faced many challenges running the household alone, getting us kids to school in the morning, fixing things that broke down in the house, and trying to budget for the many expenses of raising a family.

While my mother was worn ragged trying to manage on her own, life in Korea was not exactly a "hardship" tour for my father. He dove headlong into the Korean culture, started a teen club and a hiking club in Seoul, and befriended many young people who affectionately called him *harabaji*, or grandfather.

When my father finally returned, after being away almost two years, he restored order in our home. I sensed that his time in Korea had changed him in some way that I couldn't put my finger on. I wanted to find out what had happened over there.

Over the next few years, letters kept arriving from Korea, pasted with unusual stamps and addressed with unfamiliar handwriting. In the meantime, our family moved to Frankfurt, Germany, where my father, now a general, assumed the post of assistant division commander of the US troops stationed there.

One day, alone for the afternoon in our home in Germany, I went into my father's office to search for a pair of scissors in his dark cherry wood desk. When I saw the stacks of letters from Korea neatly crammed into the top two drawers, irresistible curiosity took hold of me. I had always wanted to know more about my father's other life in Korea. Now was my chance.

At the Pub

It's a crime to go through other people's mail. I'll beg for forgiveness if I'm caught.

The letters were poignant, each one full of appreciation and affection from young Korean men and women, thanking my father for all the many ways he had affected their lives. Among his countless acts of kindness, he had helped many students, financially and strategically, to come to the States and get a college education.

I read every word of those letters, understanding that my father had a life separate from our family—a life that apparently was quite fulfilling. The feeling of pride in my father for the difference he had made in people's lives was tinged with envy of the attention he'd given to his young Korean friends.

After completing the Korean correspondence, I began the next pile, a small stack of letters written in German with careful and deliberate handwriting, and signed by "Edith Zschiesche."

I didn't read beyond the first few perfume-scented letters. I was too stunned and sick at heart. In the first letter I learned that my father and Frau Zschiesche had been meeting while my father was overseeing military maneuvers in Grafenwoehr, near the German border with Czechoslovakia. She referred to the fun they'd had *unter der daune Decke*—under the eiderdown quilt. Shock and betrayal hit me in the solar plexus like a compressed air gun, followed by a wave of sadness for my mother. I vowed I would never tell her, although I suspected she might have somehow sensed his infidelity.

When my father came home from work that evening, I made sure to avoid him. If our paths crossed, I looked away. He asked what was wrong. I told him, "I hate you, Daddy. I'm never going to speak to you again." My pronouncement was no small matter, given our history of being best buddies.

For the following week, I didn't speak a word to him. He was perplexed and hurt by my behavior. Eventually, he must have seen that his letters had been tampered with.

He cornered me one day after a week of my silent treatment and asked if we could have a talk. He said he wanted to take me out for a beer. I was 16 at the time, in my junior year of high school. The invitation to drink a beer with my own father outweighed my anger. I agreed.

We drove to the local pub in downtown Frankfurt. We sat on bar stools at a little round table and sipped our beers. I didn't like the taste, but I drank it anyway because it seemed to be symbolic of our truce and a grown-up thing to do.

The conversation began awkwardly. It wasn't until my father was on his second beer that his talk came more freely. Without ever acknowledging my discovery of his secret affair, he said, "Rickie, you have to understand how difficult it's been living with your mother. She's rejecting and critical of everything I do. We haven't had sex since John was born 13 years ago."

Whoa! I can't handle this.

I felt my face flush with embarrassment. I tilted my head down towards my beer stein so my father wouldn't see how uncomfortable I was hearing him talk about his and my mother's sex life, or lack thereof.

He continued, "A man needs to feel loved. I'm starving for some affection from your mother."

My anger softened with each revelation. Although I was in deep water—way over my teenage head in this role as confidante to my father—I felt sorry for him and realized that I had put him on a pedestal and expected him to be perfect. Even though I adored him, I got a flash of insight that he was just a regular guy who needed affection—not that different from me.

"Rickie, can you forgive me?"

"Of course I can, Daddy," I said, trying to sound reassuring, hoping he wouldn't notice my inner ambivalence, revulsion, and confusion.

It was painful listening to my father talk about sex, a Merriam family taboo. No one talked about this subject in my family.

When my father and I returned home from the pub, I went to my room and cried, releasing my pent-up hurt and anger from the prior week. My tears were for my mother, too, for the deception she was living with. I wondered if she knew my father was unfaithful. I wondered if she recognized that she wasn't giving him what he needed, and if so, did she accept that he would go elsewhere to meet his needs? I didn't dare ask her.

I wanted to protect my mother from my father's betrayal—and his dissatisfaction—which would surely shatter her world. After all, she had lost her parents at a tender age and had never received adequate affection. She showed her love through her devoted attention to our physical wellbeing—keeping us in freshly washed and ironed clothes, feeding us healthy foods, and keeping a well-scoured house. Even the harsh discipline she dispensed demonstrated her version of love, which she must have learned as a child in Switzerland from her stern and often cruel stepmothers—two of them over the course of her childhood.

My mother was only six years old when her mother bled to death from a ruptured tubal pregnancy. Her beloved father was rarely present, constantly on duty as the town's only doctor. She had no one to protect her from the cruelty of her consecutive stepmothers.

When her father died of pneumonia, my mother became a virtual orphan when she was 16 years old.

I grieved not only for my mother. I grieved for my loss too—the loss of the idealized image I had of my father. As that image receded, I felt myself entering uncharted territory, where old feelings were giving way to new ones. Over time, my need to view people as all bad or all good, villains or heroes, evolved into a kind of acceptance that could encompass human flaws as well as sterling traits, especially in those I loved.

After I told this story to Dr. Samuels, I mentioned that my new way of seeing the world was being put to the test all too frequently. He wanted me to explain what exactly I meant by that statement. I told him about my father's shocking reaction to my first attempt to look pretty.

Chapter 9

CUTTING THE BRAID

Frankfurt, Germany, 1965

My long braid hit the floor with the dull thud of a severed limb. This part of me was gone—forever. I knew my life would never be the same.

A few seconds of regret washed over me.

Oh geez. What have I done?

"Don't worry. You can sell it to a wig maker for a lot of money," Karen said from behind me.

Karen lived across the street from us in the enclave of military families stationed in Frankfurt, Germany. We both had just begun our senior year of high school. We were the same age, but Karen exuded a juicy sensuality and sophistication that I admired.

One Sunday afternoon, Karen invited me over. Not long into the visit, she began educating me about the benefits of makeup and asked if I would like her to give me a makeover. After a few seconds of hesitation, I agreed.

I sat at her vanity table, which was covered with brushes, eyeliner pencils, lipsticks, jars of powders, a tray of eye shadow colors, and a little sponge. I closed my eyes and waited in suspense while she painted my face.

When I opened my eyes, the newly made-up face looking back at me from the vanity mirror was fascinating and pretty—in an artificial way—with no resemblance to anyone in my family.

"You look great, Rickie. Don't you just love your new look?"

"I think so. I'm not really sure. I'll have to get used to it."

"Hey, I have a good idea," Karen continued. "Why don't we cut your hair? That braid down your back makes you look like a German schoolgirl. You'd look really sexy with short hair. We could curl it up into a flip or curl it under into a pageboy. I'll go get my mom's scissors."

"No! Wait a minute. Umm… Let me think about it."

My father liked my long braid, probably because it made me look like a tomboy. And my younger brother John had said, in a moment of sibling revenge, that my long, thick hair was the only thing I had going for me.

John and I were creative at getting revenge on each other, although we were quite bonded due to our isolation in Germany. We missed our four older siblings, who were in college, graduate school, or working. And we missed our civilian friends back in the States.

At 16, the year before my visit with Karen, I'd had innocent crushes on a motley assortment of boys. Yet, at the same time I was painfully shy when boys started relating to me as a sexual being rather than as their buddy on the playing field or their partner in the high school chemistry lab.

One afternoon after school, while my parents were away, John yelled that there was a boy coming to the house to visit me. I peeked out the living room window and saw Danny walking toward the front door. He was a big guy, a star on the football team. He had recently started sitting next to me in the cafeteria, exuding an interest that made me ill at ease. I had no idea what to talk to him about. I dove into the hall closet opposite the front door to hide.

"Johnny, tell Danny I'm not home."

"How much will you pay me to tell him that?"

"Fifty cents."

He warned me that fifty cents wasn't enough for telling a lie. He would only do it for a dollar. There wasn't time to negotiate as John opened the door to let Danny in.

"Is your sister home?"

"Yes, she is. She's hiding right here in the closet."

Karen's hypnotic voice interrupted my thoughts. Her words painted a picture of glamour and romantic possibilities once I was freed from the braid. In my hypnotized state, I agreed to let her cut it off. I closed my eyes, not wanting to watch the amputation.

Within a few minutes, I heard the thump. On the floor next to my chair lay the long, thick brown braid—my only asset—now a lifeless corpse.

Karen reassured me that the braid had needed to come off. After she finished trimming my hair, curling it in hot rollers, and dousing it in hair spray, I stared into the mirror at the new me, feeling ecstatic, fascinated, and uncomfortable all at the same time—not quite certain about stepping into this new version of me. I wondered what my parents would think.

While Karen performed the finishing touches on her bouffant-style creation, I asked, "What do you talk about when you're with boys? I never know what to say to them."

"If you want to get a boy to talk, just ask about football, or baseball, or cars," she said knowingly.

"But I don't know anything about those things, and I'm not really interested in them either."

"That doesn't matter," she explained. "Just pretend you're interested."

By the time Karen finished with my total makeover, it was nighttime. I crossed the street to my home, excited to show my parents my new look. They had just returned from a few days of visiting relatives in Switzerland and were sitting at the dining room table eating dinner when I walked in and greeted them enthusiastically.

Dead silence.

My mother looked me over. Then her voice shattered the silence. "What did you do to your hair?"

Before I could answer, my father stood up stiffly from the head of the table. "You look like a whore," he growled. He picked up his antique chair and slammed it down with such force that one of the legs splintered in half. He stormed upstairs to his bedroom.

Hurt and confused, I too stormed up to my room and slammed the door with all the force I had. I threw myself on my bed and cried. The makeup pooled on my pillow and smudged my face.

How could he say such a horrible thing to me?

I didn't understand what was going on. It appeared I had broken some big, unspoken taboo about looking attractive. I flashed back to a long-forgotten memory from the mid-1950s. My family was waiting in a hotel room to board the ship that would take us back to the States from England, where we had been living for three years. I was six. My 15-year-old sister, Vreni, had put lipstick on for the first time. My father told her to take it off. She said no. He insisted and she refused, whereupon he slapped her so hard, she fell to the ground. He didn't tell her what was wrong with wearing lipstick.

I had never seen my father hit anyone before, other than the spankings we all got routinely. I had a difficult time integrating this violent scene with my adoration of him as a peacemaker, a man of great kindness. The only way I could resolve the discrepancy was to push the incident out of my mind entirely.

While remembering other incidents from the past, struggling to make meaning out of the outburst that had just occurred downstairs, I heard a rustling of paper outside my bedroom. And then a folded piece of paper appeared under the door. The note said, "I'm sorry. Sometimes fathers have trouble understanding their daughters."

The cutting of the braid and the makeup were never spoken of again. But the incident left me with the unarticulated feeling that looking too pretty might be dangerous.

Dangerous for whom? For me? For my father?

It was all terribly confusing. I thought about the times my father would not let any of his daughters give him a massage, even a shoulder massage. I wondered if this was some kind of clue to what had just happened.

Taking into account my childhood history of being my father's buddy, it dawned on me that he was probably grieving over my transition to becoming a woman and leaving behind our years of being buddies.

I was ambivalent myself about becoming a woman. At 13, I started changing in ways I didn't fully understand. There were no sex education classes in those days. Parents were supposed to teach their children about these delicate matters, but none of my family members or even friends wanted to speak about the subject. I was ignorant about bodily functions related to pleasure and procreation, and I didn't really have any interest in the subject until I was well into my teen years. I did hear a rumor going around that girls could get pregnant if they kissed in a certain way. I assumed that meant if the tongue was involved.

When I got my first period, I had no idea why there was blood in my underwear. I told my mother I had gotten cut somehow. The topic of menstruation had never been addressed with me. She gave me an explanation about the blood that I only vaguely understood.

She warned me about boys, "You are a woman now, Rickie. That means that you could get pregnant. You need to be very careful around boys. All they're interested in is sex." She handed me a box of pads and told me to wear them the next time I bled. That was the end of the conversation. The topic clearly made her uncomfortable.

My older sister Susie talked to me a bit about what was happening, but it all sounded so disgusting. I envied boys. I thought they got a better deal. Becoming a woman did not seem like much fun if it meant you had to bleed every month and worry about getting pregnant.

In spite of my initial ambivalence during puberty about being female, the cutting of the braid symbolized freedom to explore my new role as a young woman. Although I felt some sadness about stepping out of the role of being best buddies with my father, I surprised myself as I embraced my transition into womanhood better than I ever could have imagined.

Chapter 10

CUTTING LOOSE

Frankfurt, Germany, early spring 1966

After Karen cut off my braid, my life as a senior high school student radically changed. I felt as though I had become a different person.

The student body at Frankfurt American High School chose me to "man" the kissing booth, a plan that came from a school-wide brainstorming session on ways to raise money to replace the football team's worn-out equipment.

> *Yikes! They want ME to kiss the boys? Why me? I wonder if it's related to cutting off the braid and looking more like a woman.*

The idea scared me, but that made it all the more intriguing. I liked to take on a challenge to see if I had the nerve to do it. When my high school girlfriends painted my face with heavy makeup and dressed me in black mesh stockings, a push-up bra, and low-cut blouse, I was counting on my love of theater and mimicking others to help me overcome my fear and lack of confidence with boys.

I looked like one of the flirtatious barmaids at the local pub in downtown Frankfurt, a far cry from a general's daughter. The risk of being caught by my parents, who expected me to set a good example at all times, increased the thrill.

The boys stood in line to get their dollar's worth at the kissing booth. I shut my eyes and held my breath with each kiss, hoping it would be quick—and hoping I was convincing in the role of a girl who enjoyed kissing a queue of boys. Thankfully, the kisses were quick, with lips closed tight.

In a black-and-white photograph, documented for all posterity, one can see my tightly clenched left hand, the telltale sign of my determination to succeed in my mission to raise money—and of my discomfort.

> *Why did I agree to do this? If a girl kisses a boy for money, does that mean she's a whore? Is she a whore even if the money is for a good cause?*

Being part of a family that moved every couple years or so, I had grown up learning how to be accepted by each new group of classmates in each new environment and culture. I faced my first big challenge in England at age six when my teacher urged me to drop my "Yankee accent" and enunciate clearly like a well-educated Brit. I quickly discovered that to look, speak, and act like the people around you is key to making new friends and avoiding ridicule. I acquired quite a talent for mimicking people.

By the time I kissed the last boy in line at the kissing booth—my mission completed—I wasn't ready to end the performance. My heart was racing from all the kissing. My body overflowed with surges of adrenaline that needed an outlet. I impulsively jumped onto a cafeteria table that had been set up under the big party tent and, with shameless exuberance, sang in the deepest Marlene Dietrich voice I could manage, "Hey look me over, lend me an ear, fresh out of clover, mortgage up to here…"

Mercifully, no one told my parents about my improper behavior.

Unbeknownst to me, the director of the drama department stood under the party tent watching my spontaneous performance. He recognized my love of acting and invited me to audition for a part in the senior play, *Bye Bye Birdie*.

I got the role of Albert's mother, Mae Peterson. I took on the personality of a high-strung, long-suffering martyr with a heavy Brooklyn accent, desperately manipulative in order to get her son's attention and resentful of his girlfriend. I loved every minute of playing this role.

But acting in the kissing booth and then in front of an audience were just the first stages of my newfound liberation that spring of my senior year.

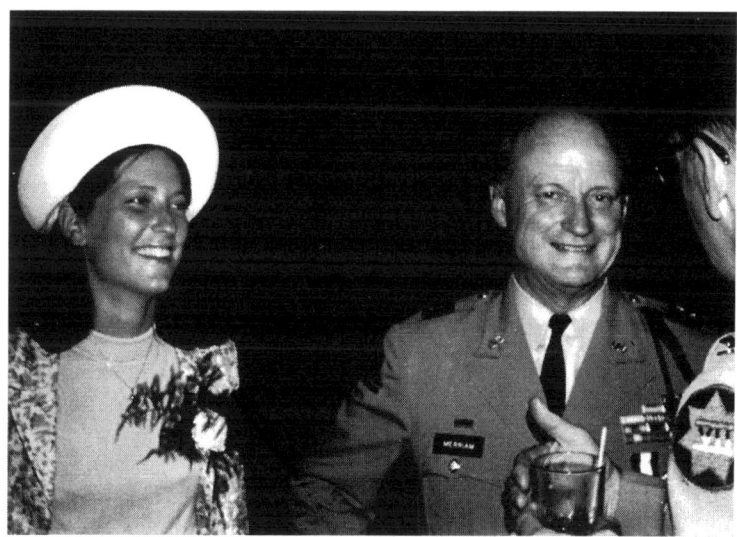

By the time I attended my father's retirement ceremony, I had already stepped into my new role as a young woman, which I learned to enjoy more than I could have imagined.

Chapter 11

JEAN PIERRE

As I recounted to Dr. Samuels the stories of my earlier life, he listened attentively. Sometimes I saw him press his lips together as though he were trying to suppress a smile. In one session, he asked me to talk about my first sexual experience. He thought it might shed light on the forces at play in my life, especially while I explored my new role as a young woman.

I first met Jean Pierre when I was 12 years old. He was a close friend of my older sister, Jackie, who had spent her junior year abroad studying at the Sorbonne in Paris. Jean Pierre was like a brother to her. The year after Jackie returned home to the States, Jean Pierre decided to come meet our whole family.

His visit left little impression on me beyond his hilariously thick French accent, which I delighted in imitating. He was 19 at the time, and as far as I was concerned, that was old.

Four years later, my family moved to Frankfurt. Jean Pierre's mother and my mother had kept in touch over the years, ever since his visit to the States. When I was 17, the mothers hatched a plan for me to spend the spring break of my senior year in Paris at Jean Pierre's home.

Spring break arrived in no time. Jean Pierre met me at the Gare du Nord train station, as our mothers had arranged. I felt instantly attracted to him, even though he was way older than me—an "older man" at 24.

Dr. Samuels asked, "Did the mothers try to set you up?" It sure looked that way, but at the time it didn't cross my mind.

Jean Pierre gave me a grand tour of Paris, ending at the front desk of the tiny hotel I had chosen in the Latin Quarter. I preferred the freedom of a hotel to the strictures of staying in Jean Pierre's home, which I assumed meant acting like a refined young lady to meet his parents' high standards of propriety.

Jean Pierre came to visit me every day. He gazed deep into my eyes for long moments at a time. I barely breathed from embarrassment, shyness, and excitement as my eyes darted around, trying to avoid his penetrating blue-eyed gaze. I laughed with discomfort and delight.

He took me home to meet his family. I discovered that my French-speaking skills were quite adequate—a relief to me, since the older Parisians were famously critical of foreigners who attempted to speak their language.

At the end of the vacation, I left Paris with stars in my eyes and electricity in my body. As we were waiting in the train station, just before the train to Germany arrived, Jean Pierre reached over and held my face in his hands. We kissed. It was the first passionately juicy kiss I had ever experienced. I held my breath for the duration of the kissing but loved every second of it. Reluctantly, I pulled myself away as the whistle blew and the train slowly began rolling down the tracks. I ran after it and jumped on board.

During the trip back home, I relived the kissing in my mind. Jean Pierre's kisses were very different from the quick, peck-like kisses I got from the boys on the football team.

Even the drabness of high school back in Frankfurt was tolerable while I indulged in fantasies of my first potential affair. When my parents left for the evening, I pulled out my collection of French records and played them over and over, belting out the words of Édith Piaf from the depths of my teenage heart. In the late afternoons, I lay in the tall pasture grass under the old apple tree behind our house, daydreaming about my time with Jean Pierre.

The rest of senior year passed quickly. I could hardly focus on my studies anymore. My mind was on a distant horizon of possibilities.

In June of 1966 I graduated from Frankfurt American High School. My graduation coincided with my father's retirement from the army. An impressive ceremony marked the event, with hundreds of people in makeshift bleachers, a brass band, a parade, and endless speeches. High honors and medals were bestowed, along with a letter from President Johnson commending my father for his distinguished service in the military.

My parents invited Jean Pierre to attend this milestone in our Merriam family history. He arrived a few days early. His presence in our house so completely excited me that I could do nothing but grin like an imbecile. When Jean Pierre looked at me, I felt so flustered, I had to look away or down at the floor.

Jean Pierre had only intended to stay for a couple of days because my parents had planned a family trip after my father's retirement ceremony. It would be a farewell visit to places in Normandy on the northern coast of France, including the beach where my father had landed during World War II on D-Day plus two.

I asked if Jean Pierre could join us on our farewell journey. My parents agreed. Along the way, we picnicked in the French countryside and listened to my father's intriguing and sometimes gripping war stories.

On our way back home, we dropped Jean Pierre off in Paris. His parting words to me were, *On se verra bientôt.* (We'll see each other soon.) His words puzzled me.

> *How can we see each other soon? I'll be leaving for college at the end of the summer. I wonder what he means.*

A few months before graduating from high school, I had decided to spend the summer studying painting and art history in Florence, Italy, before starting college in the States in the fall of that year.

While I took painting classes and studied Renaissance art at the university, I still had plenty of time to explore Florence. As I sauntered through the streets, a bevy of young men followed close behind. At first I found the attention flattering and dared to entertain the possibility that maybe I was more attractive than I realized. Those inflated thoughts rapidly evaporated when I observed how the paparazzi whistled at and followed any foreign female between the ages of 15 and 50. From then on, the attention became annoying.

While wandering around in a museum, I struck up a conversation with a friendly Florentine man who was probably twice my age. He invited me to join him for dinner at a famous restaurant. I loved the idea of eating a big, delicious meal and accepted his invitation. I thanked him profusely for his generosity. I had grown weary of eating bread, pasta, and a salad every day, which was all I could afford with my small stipend that had to last the entire summer.

After we ordered from the menu, the man began describing what would happen after dinner, including driving me to his house in his Ferrari and having sex all night. At first, I pretended I didn't fully understand what he was saying due to my limited Italian. Then he switched to broken English and gave the same description of what he was going to do with me. Terrified, I told him I had never had sex before and that I was faithful to my French boyfriend. He wasn't fazed in the least. He talked as though the invitation to dinner was part of an unspoken business deal and that I had to keep my end of the bargain.

Oh God! How do I get out of this mess?

I excused myself and said that I had to use the bathroom. As I pondered what to do, I saw a large casement window above the toilet. I cranked the window open as far as I could, hoisted my legs through the window while holding onto a pipe for support, and then wiggled the rest of my body out the window and jumped to the ground and landed on a patch of grass in a back alley. I ran as fast as I could back to my host family's house.

Learning how to be a young woman around men was a steep learning curve. I'd never faced these challenges when I had my braid. But once I caught on to some of the unspoken rules of the male-female game, I learned quickly.

In August I received a telegram from Jean Pierre urging me to join him in Turkey, where he worked as an apprentice in international banking in the city of Izmir. A few days later, a plane ticket came in the mail. I packed my blue suitcase and said goodbye to Florence, promising myself to return someday to this enchanting place.

When I arrived in Izmir's tiny airport, Jean Pierre was nowhere to be seen. I waited. And I waited. Maybe he had not received my telegram telling him of the change in my arrival date due to my final exam schedule.

I had no idea where Jean Pierre lived or worked. To make matters worse, I couldn't find my suitcase in baggage claim and learned that it had been misplaced in Athens during the change of planes. As insurance, I picked up the remaining bag that had not been claimed. It was also blue and looked identical to mine. I figured it would give me more bargaining power in getting my own back. Beyond that, it wasn't much use since it was locked.

As ten o'clock approached, the small airport terminal began to close down for the night. I assessed my situation: no money, no address, no friend, no ability to speak the language, no knowledge whatsoever about Muslim countries. Not good.

I found a man behind one of the counters who spoke a little English and asked if he could help me. He listened to my plight attentively. He said there was a US Air Force base in town where I might get help from my compatriots. He pointed to a bus idling outside that would be leaving for the base in a few minutes. I hopped on board.

To my relief, I found several American soldiers on the bus. I picked out one with a compassionate face and sat down next to him. When he heard my story, he took me to a hotel and bought me a room.

> *I wonder if he's expecting something sexual from me in return? Oh God, I'll have to think up some way to avoid this.*

I did some fast talking, saying I'd traveled to Izmir because Jean Pierre and I planned to get married. Soon it became apparent there was no need for pretense. The soldier gave me pure kindness, with no price attached.

The next day I got in touch with the police department and asked for help in tracking down Jean Pierre. My generous Air Force benefactor came to visit me for a couple hours to offer moral support. The rest of the time I spent roaming around the city alone.

Izmir, a beautiful port city bordering the Aegean Sea with mountains in the background, dates back to 3,000 BC. The legendary Homer lived there in the Greek Ionian period when it was called

Smyrna. I walked along the palm-lined boulevards, watched the ships and yachts bobbing in the bay, listened to the periodic calls to worship emanating from loudspeakers in the minarets, passed tea shops with intoxicating smells of spices, and wandered through bazaars selling exotic goods.

I felt both fascinated and frightened by the strange people and sights. The men who passed me in the street looked at me as though I had no clothes on. The women, covered in headscarves, just looked away. I saw myself for the first time through their eyes—a young American woman, scantily clad in a flimsy Florentine blouse and a brightly colored miniskirt that only covered three-quarters of her thighs, walking alone, without a man.

I became unbearably self-conscious. I had come to Turkey in an era long before easy international travel filled the city's streets with tourists from around the world, clad in various styles of immodest clothing.

Since my below-the-knee-length skirts and pants lay neatly folded up in my errant suitcase in Athens, it seemed safer for me to return to the hotel and stay in hiding.

Meanwhile, Jean Pierre had received my telegram a day late. He too had put himself in touch with the police in an effort to locate me. After three days, we finally made contact. We were overjoyed to find each other. Our reunion was poignant and thrilling.

After we managed to pull ourselves apart, Jean Pierre grabbed my hand and led me to one of the main banks, right in the heart of the city, where he apprenticed with Turkish banking officials.

We passed his office on the first floor and headed up the stairs to his tiny apartment on the third floor. Windows lined one wall with a view overlooking the Aegean Sea.

Jean Pierre

Jean Pierre and I spent that evening romancing in bed. After a while, he told me to take off all my clothes so we could take a shower together. I felt terribly embarrassed and shy—and a bit frightened.

After the shower, we rolled around together in the bed, arms and legs twisted among the sheets. Jean Pierre was passionate. I felt like a scared observer. This was uncharted territory for me.

I felt some strange sensations—some of them quite painful—as he penetrated me and began making thrusting movements with his body.

> *I thought making love was supposed to feel good.*

I watched Jean Pierre while his eyes were closed tight. His face began to turn red. I couldn't tell if the contorted expressions and moaning sounds came from pain or pleasure. His breathing became faster and faster, sounding like panting. I could feel his heart racing against my chest. With all this intensity and concentration, I was positive something earthshaking was about to happen. I just hoped it wasn't a heart attack.

Unexpectedly, after some jerking movements, Jean Pierre's body became still and limp. I didn't know what was happening or why he suddenly stopped. We lay quietly embracing as my mind churned.

> *Oh my god! I've just been deflowered on the third floor of a bank in Turkey. When people see me in the street I wonder if they'll be able to recognize that I'm not a virgin. I wonder if there's some way people can tell.*

After I got beyond the stage of looking on as an objective observer and the pain that comes from losing one's virginity, I began looking forward to making love and became an enthusiastic participant. I fell madly in love with Jean Pierre. I had never felt so much joy in my whole life.

That adventurous month with Jean Pierre, in August of 1966, was a truly enchanting time for me, when I enthusiastically lost my innocence. In contrast to my tomboy years when I dreaded the thought of becoming a woman and wanted nothing to do with that part of life, I now decided that I thoroughly enjoyed my gender and would never want to trade it.

Summer slid into September and came to an end. At the train station in Paris, Jean Pierre gave me an engagement ring that was a family heirloom. As he slid the ring on my finger, he said that we were officially engaged and that we would get married when I returned for my junior year abroad.

"Rickie, tu seras toujours dans mon cœur. Je ne t'oublierai jamais. Le temps passera vite. Tu verras." Jean Pierre said he would always keep me in his heart and would never forget me. He assured me that the time would pass quickly. We had a tearful, heartrending goodbye, filled with last-minute promises.

The flight passed quickly as I sat lost in sweet reveries. My father picked me up at the Boston airport and drove me to his and my mother's new home in New Hampshire, where they had recently moved after leaving Germany. They lived near Franklin Pierce College, where my father had begun his third career in life as dean of students.

I settled in as much as possible in the short interlude before leaving for college. It was a bittersweet time for me. I was pining for Jean Pierre. Yet at the same time, without any clear understanding of what awaited me, I readied myself to cross over a threshold and leave behind the life I had known in Europe.

Chapter 12

SLAYING THE DRAGONS

Dr. Samuels said that I obviously enjoyed my new role as a woman. I agreed, but since coming to Antioch I had become a very confused young woman and an unhappy wife. On that note, Dr. Samuels wanted me to speak more about my marriage to Jeff. "Why do you think your marriage might not last?" he asked.

I thought for a minute. "Well, I'm not a very good wife. I'm too demanding. I'm never just content with the way things are."

"Do you think this might have something to do with the way you were raised?"

"I guess so. My mother was demanding. I don't think she was very happy with herself, so she took it out on her children. Maybe I'm doing the same thing with Jeff. I make him feel like he's never good enough—just what my mother did with us. And I even blame him for things that aren't really his problem. They're my problem, but I can't admit it—like blaming him for my unhappiness, claiming that he's too critical of me and then not acknowledging that I'm too critical of myself. Now that you mention it, I guess I went from feeling oppressed as a child to becoming the oppressor. What an awful thought."

Dr. Samuels abruptly changed the subject when he noticed my teeth were chattering. "I want to digress a moment. I just now noticed that you've come to this appointment *barefooted*. Erica, it's the middle of winter and there's snow on the ground. And I notice you didn't wear a coat or sweater. Is there some reason you're doing this?"

"Actually, I've been coming barefoot for the past few sessions, but you didn't notice. I'm trying to make myself strong so that I won't be so sensitive to life and things won't be so painful," I explained.

"But how will making yourself physically strong help you become emotionally strong?" he asked.

"I don't know. I just had a feeling that if I toughened up, my feelings wouldn't get hurt so easily."

"Erica, the best way to become less sensitive to what happens in life is to understand yourself better—which will help you understand others better. And that's what we're doing here in these appointments." Dr. Samuels' answer gave me a lot to think about.

He continued, "You don't need to go barefoot anymore to make your feet tough. In fact, I want you to wear shoes at our appointments. And please wear a coat.

"Now, let's get back to your marriage with Jeff and see if we can get some insights. Once you develop an understanding of the forces at work in your life, you'll no longer feel like a victim of circumstances. What other observations have you made?" he asked.

"When I cook meals for Jeff and me, I expect Jeff to rave about how amazing the meal is. When he doesn't say anything, I feel like a failure. My mother did the same thing. I guess she just wanted to feel appreciated."

When Jeff and I met, he fell madly in love with me. I got addicted to being loved in that intense way, with the frequent expressions of devotion. So, when things simmered down after we got to really know each other, I missed the passion and felt unloved. I had an insatiable hunger for affection. I think a normal person who had been raised in a loving home would just accept the fact that the initial intensity of falling in love can't last.

"I wish I were a normal person and not so defective," I said plaintively.

"You judge yourself harshly. Your mother judged you harshly as a child. You internalized the judgments—even though your mother no longer does that much anymore, according to what you've told me."

Dr. Samuels said there is no such thing as a "normal" person. Human beings are all looking for some form of love—*that's* what's normal. He explained that each of us has our own unique and all-too-often distorted ways of expressing that need based on what we learned as children. And I was young and still learning about myself and about life.

He went on to say that when children do not feel loved and nurtured by their mother, they spend much of their lives in pursuit of that love. They become a bottomless pit of need that can never be satisfied.

"No one can make up for what you didn't get from your mother. Once you understand that, you can start learning how to satisfy that need in healthy ways that are not self-defeating. I'll wager that Jeff has some unmet needs for love as well. Most people do."

We spent many sessions analyzing my behavior in the marriage. In the end, Dr. Samuels said that even if I were the most mentally healthy person on Earth, the marriage would probably still need to end simply because we were mere teenagers when we married and still undergoing major changes.

At home with Jeff, I felt a sadness coming from him. He expressed gratitude that I was seeing Dr. Samuels and trying to sort things out. Even in the face of the marital disintegration, it was obvious that we loved each other. I still regarded Jeff as my best friend and confidant. We held each other and cried a lot together. The thought of separating was unbearable, but it seemed inevitable.

Although we both knew where the marriage was heading, we didn't talk about divorce. We disguised that fear by talking about our need to explore life on our own for a few months, and then—we earnestly assured each other—we'd get back together.

During one session, Dr. Samuels asked me about my siblings. I confessed that I had a dark secret that I hadn't told anyone. My face flushed with embarrassment as I thought about revealing to him this festering fact that I had locked up inside of me. He sat in his chair with an expectant look.

"Dr. Samuels, I know you'll be shocked. You probably won't like me anymore," I said through tears, with a racing heart.

"I'm not a very intelligent person. I'm actually pretty dumb. I've just been pretending that I'm smart most of my life. I'm a good actress and have everyone convinced that I'm smart—except for my own family."

Dr. Samuels looked puzzled. "What are you talking about, Erica? Of course you're intelligent. You're highly intelligent. I read your file. You took honors courses in high school and got straight A's. I read the enthusiastic letters of recommendation that your high school teachers wrote. You're doing very well academically with excellent evaluations from your college professors. And you have the distinction of speaking several foreign languages. There's no way to fake those kinds of achievements. I think—"

I interrupted, "My sisters skipped grades because school was too easy for them. They went to college when they were sixteen and got big scholarships. My oldest sister, Vreni, is on a full scholarship studying Chinese at Harvard. My second-oldest sister, Jackie, is at

Yale on a scholarship, and my sister, Susie, scored in the top one percent on her IQ test, resulting in an invitation to join Mensa.

"As for me, I only got small scholarships for college. And I never skipped any grades. I wasn't smart enough. I had to work hard in school. My sisters could read a thick book in a day or two. It took me many days to read a book. And I never dared to take an IQ test. I didn't want to know."

My sisters were the intellectuals in the family. I was the athlete, tall and strong—with the weaker brain. My brother John liked to taunt me by calling me an "Amazon" with a tone of disdain, especially after we had physical fights that I won.

I had to look up in the Merriam-Webster dictionary what he meant by calling me an Amazon. I discovered that the word referred to mythical Greek women warriors who were big and strong. That description did not sound bad to me, but John had used the word in a derogatory way.

"Outside of my family, I somehow managed to fool everyone into thinking that I was really smart," I stated with conviction.

Dr. Samuels had a bemused look on his face. He asked me to give him examples of times when I first began feeling stupid. I had a hard time remembering specific incidents. The feelings of being stupid and not good enough pervaded my entire childhood.

After some moments of silent reflection, I remembered that John had also called me a "stupid idiot" during fights and often made fun of me, although I was no angel with him either.

I recounted a seemingly insignificant incident that happened when I was 12 years old and John was nine. I overheard him talking to one of his friends about World War II. He mentioned that he had read a history book about a war hero who was hit by shrapnel and died. I interrupted the conversation and asked John who Shrapnel was. He said that Shrapnel was a famous general in World War II and then burst out laughing and called me stupid because I hadn't heard of shrapnel. Humiliated, I asked my father if he knew General Shrapnel. He said that there was no such person and that the word shrapnel referred to fragments that fly into the air after an explosion from a bomb.

As Dr. Samuels cleared his throat, I saw him purse his lips to suppress a smile. Seeing his reaction helped me get a glimpse of the humor in my interactions with my brother.

Dr. Samuels intercepted the case I was making to convince him of my stupidity. He pointed out that children often interpret literally what is said to them. He asked me if I had ever called someone "stupid" simply out of anger or frustration—without meaning that they were literally stupid. I acknowledged that I had. In fact, I had called my brother "stupid" on quite a few occasions. But my brother never believed for a second that he was stupid.

Dr. Samuels told me that if I spent my time comparing my intellect to that of my siblings, I would overlook my own unique strengths and intelligence, and that I would never have the pleasure of appreciating who I am. He pointed out that the IQ tests only measure a certain kind of intelligence.

Because I totally trusted Dr. Samuels, I took his words to heart and considered the possibility that I might be genuinely intelligent after all—in my own unique way.

Chapter 13

MY MOTHER AND ME

IN SOME OF THE SESSIONS, Dr. Samuels wanted to focus on my relationship with my mother. When I told him that my mother's name was Erica, he asked me if I resembled her in any way. At the time, I was not able to see even a remote resemblance. It was a mystery to me why my parents had given my mother's name to me, the fifth out of six children.

Dr. Samuels asked me to describe my mother. "Mummy has black hair and green eyes," I told him. "She's slender, with high cheekbones and fine features—not the blonde, robust Swiss stereotype. Her ancestors were French Huguenots who fled to Switzerland in the 1700s to avoid religious persecution. She's proud of that lineage. She speaks with a soft foreign accent and prides herself on having learned 'proper' English in England.

"Mummy is beautiful, cultured, intelligent, chronically worried about everything, and impossibly critical. She ran our household in the strict style of old Europe, where hitting and slapping her children was 'for our own good.'"

Although I got high praise from my teachers at school, at home I got the message that I wasn't good enough, no matter how hard I tried.

My mother was so musically gifted, she couldn't fathom why I made so many mistakes as I was learning to play the piano. She thought I was playing the wrong notes on purpose to irritate her. She reacted by whacking the side of my head with the palm of her hand. Any traces of musical abilities in me were aborted around that time.

In college, I tried to resuscitate my musical life by taking piano lessons with an endlessly patient teacher who taught elementary school kids. Once when the teacher reached over to turn the page, the movement of her hand in my peripheral vision triggered some ancient cellular memory of being hit from the side by my mother. I reflexively cowered with my hands over my head. The teacher looked thoroughly bemused. All I could do was laugh with embarrassment.

My mother did a superb job attending to our physical needs, but she did not know how to address our emotional lives. We were supposed to be tough and not complain. We were alone in the uncharted wilderness of our inner worlds, trying to make sense out of our feelings.

My mother's father was the town doctor—a kind man, but always busy taking care of his patients. She didn't see him much even though the clinic occupied the entire ground floor of their mansion.

What my mother and her younger brother Ernst endured at the hands of their stepmothers sounded to me like something from Grimms' Fairy Tales and would today be called child abuse.

Dr. Samuels pored over the family photographs that I had brought in at his request. "You have a very handsome family," he said. "Your mother clearly looks European. She seems so refined and glamorous in this one taken before she came to America. There's no clue in any of these photographs about the heartless childhood she had in Switzerland. But it came out in the way she mothered you and your siblings. The hitting, blaming, and harsh criticism."

The work of raising six children left her with frayed nerves most of the time. I wondered why she had so many children. I think even one child would have been a lot for her temperament.

We all asked ourselves why she never hired help with cleaning and cooking. Mummy was a perfectionist, a state of mind that leads to perpetual discontent. No help was good enough for her—whether paid help or help from her children. We were criticized if we didn't pitch in, and then criticized if we did try and the results were anything less than perfect. We couldn't win. "I work myself to the bone," she would say to us with recrimination in her voice.

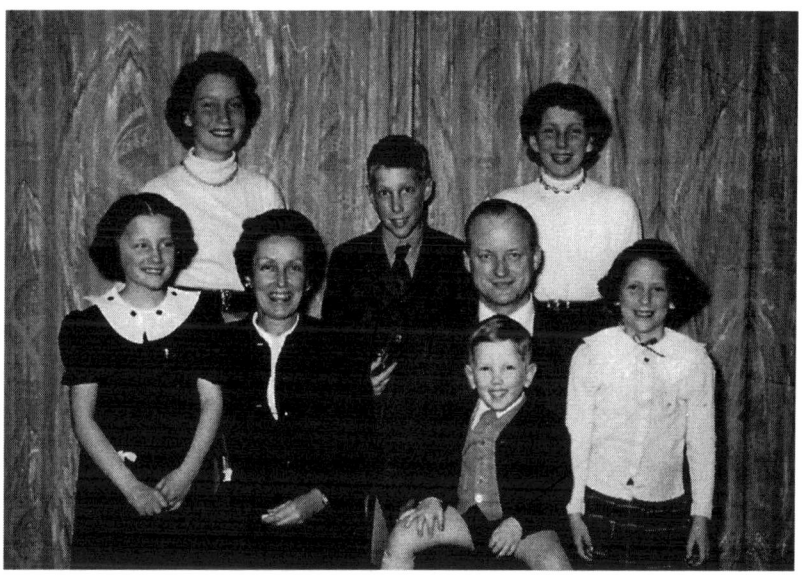

This family portrait was taken in England in 1954.
I'm in the front row on the right, age six. John is sitting on my father's lap, age three. Susie (now known as Veet), age eight, is standing next to my mother. In back are my older siblings:
Vreni, George, and Jackie.

Ironically, she came from an upper-class background; her family had servants. She went from that kind of upbringing to scrubbing her own floors. It's as though she were trying to prove something to someone, or to herself.

Mummy did have some tender moments, but they were unpredictable. A favorite memory I have of my mother involved a big freckle on one of my forearms. I didn't like it and wanted flawless skin like my friends at school. One day, in an unexpected tender moment with her, I confided that I didn't like the freckle. She put me on her lap and looked over my arms carefully and said that the freckles were beautiful. Such a statement from my mother was so unusual. I held onto it as proof to myself that my mother's real nature, behind all the harshness and criticism, was tender and loving.

We got glimpses of this side of her on the rare occasions when she was relaxed. My father sometimes offered her a glass of wine in the evenings, probably with the intention of seeing her unwind. She usually refused, knowing how easily she became intoxicated and out of control, even after just a tiny amount. But on the occasions when she did swallow a sip or two of wine, all the tension left her. She became utterly charming and looked beautiful. In those moments, it was easy to see why my father had fallen in love with her.

Dr. Samuels asked what it was like having a foreign mother growing up. I felt embarrassed by my mother's accent, especially when we moved back to the States after living in England for three years. I entered second grade in a small town in Texas after the school year had begun. When I walked into the classroom, all the students turned around and stared at me. When they heard me speak with a foreign accent, one of the boys asked me if I was a Communist. I had no idea what a Communist was, but from the tone of his voice, I knew I needed to adamantly deny the accusation. Much later, I learned about the McCarthy-era hysteria over Communism.

I started imitating the drawl of Texas speech, dragging out the vowels and slurring my words. I practiced in front of the mirror at home. I had already been exposed to several foreign languages. Texas talk was simply another one. I quickly dropped the precise enunciation that my teachers urged me to learn at school in England. Above all else, I wanted to fit in and avoid being an object of curiosity and mean-spirited teasing.

I worried about the school finding out that my mother had a foreign accent. I tore up the school's PTA notices we were supposed to give our parents for the quarterly parent/teacher meetings. It was bad enough dealing with my own accent. I never invited anyone to play at my house; I already felt different enough and didn't need to add to my problems.

"Have you always felt you were different?" Dr. Samuels asked.

Ever since I was little, I've felt different from other people. Maybe that's because of living in so many places and not really belonging anywhere. I have a different perspective on life than the people I went to school with. I question everything that others take for granted. I notice things they don't see or think about.

At the various schools I attended, each group of kids I hung out with—the nerds, the rebels, the social butterflies, and the athletes—thought I was one of them. I fit in everywhere I went—and yet I didn't really belong anywhere. I felt like an imposter.

"After spending so many years adapting to my surroundings, sometimes I wonder who I really am," I said.

Dr. Samuels sucked on his pipe, nodding as though he was pondering my words. I wondered if he'd felt the same way, like an imposter, when he got his medical degree at the University of Zurich.

"Dr. Samuels, on a different note, I just want to say before we end that I've also had—and still have—a strong feeling that there is a purpose to my life, but I have no idea what it is or how to find it. Sometimes I feel so lost. But since I've been talking to you, things are starting to make more sense."

"Before you can find your purpose in life, you need to discover who you really are. That's what these sessions are all about. It's time to wrap up. As usual, we've gone far over the hour. That's why I always schedule our session at the end of the day."

"I'm so sorry to make you late, Dr. Samuels."

"Why do you apologize? You haven't done anything wrong," he assured me.

I usually assume that when something isn't right, it's my fault. I grew up saying "I'm sorry" for everything. It was a never-ending refrain. I think it's because in my family we were constantly being blamed. Saying "I'm sorry" just became a habit, a reflex. In fact, I would say "I'm sorry" when someone accidentally bumped into me in the hall, as though it were my fault. When I was young, I even said I was sorry when I got sick.

"Tell me a bit about that before we wrap up. I'll take responsibility for being late," he assured me.

My mother said we got sick because we had done something wrong, like not wearing our rubber boots when it was raining, or staying up reading too late at night under the covers with a flashlight, or refusing to take our cod liver oil.

Being sick in our family was not much fun. Instead of getting loving care, ginger ale, ice cream, bedside stories, and time with the TV, we got reprimands. I remember one time waking up sick with a fever. There was no way I was going to reveal that to my mother. I pinched my cheeks to make them look rosy red—not realizing my face was already red—and went off to school.

The teacher saw my flushed face and congestion and right away recognized that I was sick. She called my mother and told her to come get me and keep me at home when I was sick. It took me years to understand that my mother's anger was masking a fear that she might lose one of her children to sickness. At least, that's the explanation I gave myself.

In spite of my mother's harsh response to sickness, I was comforted as I lay sick in bed listening to the sounds in the house—the vacuum cleaner rhythmically going back and forth, the washing machine tumbling the clothes around, the dishes clinking in the sink, and the cupboards closing in the kitchen. Those sounds had a soothing effect on me.

Dr. Samuels looked at his watch for a minute, then looked over at me and said something that took me by surprise. "I've missed my dinner. But that's okay. I really don't mind. I'd rather be here with you." My breathing became shallow as his words hung in the air.

Dr. Samuels went on to say that he no longer enjoyed spending time with his wife. He complained that she had gained so much weight that he had lost his sexual attraction to her.

Suddenly the roles were switched. As my heart pounded in my chest, I asked hesitantly, "Have you talked to your wife about how you're feeling?" He told me that he had insisted she lose weight or he would leave her. He seemed surprised that his warnings made no difference and she continued to gain weight.

I was stunned. Dr. Samuels was sharing his personal problems with me. I didn't know the protocol for therapists interacting with patients, but I knew that I felt really uncomfortable and wanted to change the subject immediately. I wanted to pretend that he never said anything about his sex life and his surprisingly harsh judgment of his wife. I felt terribly sorry for her. I mumbled that I had to leave because I needed to get some reading done before class the next day.

I wondered if every time I saw Dr. Samuels I would imagine him thinking about sex. I dreaded returning to therapy. But he never brought up his personal life again. We both acted as if nothing had happened.

A few months into the therapy, little twinges of attraction to Dr. Samuels surfaced into my awareness—but I didn't want to admit it to myself. I felt confused.

> *I can't be attracted to Dr. Samuels. I'm married and he's my psychiatrist. Maybe if I ignore these feelings, they'll go away.*

In the following sessions we discussed the hitting that went on in my family.

I told Dr. Samuels how I grew up thinking that hitting was a normal part of raising children and that it happened to everybody, especially in military families. But when I saw how differently some of my friends' parents treated their children, I realized that hitting was not necessarily something I had to accept. I started to fight back.

I was probably the most rebellious and outspoken of all the children in my family, but behind my anger and loud protests was a deep longing for my mother's love and approval. I wanted to be "good enough" in her eyes.

I loved my mother, and I also hated her at times and felt angry toward her. The anger and hatred made me feel guilty and sad. At Sunday school we read from the Bible, "Love and honor thy father and mother."

When I was a young girl, I kneeled at the edge of my bed at night with my hands clasped, looking up at the ceiling. I prayed fervently, "God, help me to be nice to Mummy." I wanted to be a good person and act loving toward her. But much of the time I wished I had a mother like my friends' mothers. They were kind and loving—or so it seemed.

When a teacher told my mother at a parent-teacher meeting that I was a smart student with a sweet disposition and a desire to be helpful to others, my mother told me she wondered if the teacher was talking about someone else.

Eventually the hitting came to an end as we grew older. In fact, after we moved to Germany when I was 16, Mummy began to treat me as her confidante, telling me how frustrated she was with my father, describing in great detail his shortcomings and all the ways she was disappointed and annoyed by him.

Dr. Samuels questioned, "You had said that your father also confided in you. How did that feel to be caught in the middle?"

I had two feelings about that. I was flattered that they turned to me to share their troubles. It made me feel important and useful. But at the same time, it made me feel really uncomfortable. They each seemed to be trying to turn me against the other so I would take sides. And then they sometimes spoke about sexual matters that were way beyond what I felt comfortable with, especially since I couldn't even imagine my parents having sex in the first place. In any case, I didn't have a clue what I was supposed to do with what they told me, so I just comforted them and listened.

Dr. Samuels asked, "What long-term effect do you think it had on you to be put in that position of being confidante to both parents?"

I think it helped me to see that there are always two sides to the story. If I had just listened to my mother, I would think that my father was a bad person. And if I just listened to my father, I would feel sorry for him and wonder why he stayed with my mother. So it helped me get the bigger picture and not get into who's right and who's wrong. And it made me realize that I can love people who are not perfect—including people like myself who are flawed.

At our next session, Dr. Samuels wanted to return to the topic of my marriage with Jeff. He inquired about my sex life and wanted to know if the way I was raised impacted my ability to enjoy sex. He wanted to know all the details of our sex life, like how many times in a day and in a week we had sex, who came first, and what positions we got into. He asked if I enjoyed having sex and asked if I ever masturbated. He said that masturbation was a good way to relax.

I confessed to Dr. Samuels that I felt really uncomfortable talking about those subjects with him. What I didn't confess to Dr. Samuels was my suspicion that he was getting pleasure from hearing about my sexual experiences. Because I put so much trust in him, it took a couple of sessions before this insight became apparent to me.

Dr. Samuels dutifully dropped the subject and never brought it up again.

His next statement took me by surprise. He said that he could detect that I was having some mixed emotions toward him. His directness disarmed me.

"I actually think I'm falling in love with you, Dr. Samuels," I blurted out and then quickly looked away. A long, uncomfortable silence followed.

Dr. Samuels cleared his throat and explained in a professorial tone that what I was experiencing was called "transference," which was a normal aspect of the doctor-patient relationship and could be therapeutic. I had indeed confused the feelings of profound gratitude for his help with a more physical kind of love.

Dr. Samuels didn't say anything about his own "counter-transference," a term that I'd learned in my freshman psychology class.

Chapter 14

BREAKTHROUGH

Spring 1970

THE FOLLOWING WEEK I TRAVELED HOME on spring break without Jeff to see my parents in New Hampshire. One evening, I was washing the dishes in the kitchen sink when I had an awakening that seemed to occur out of nowhere. Suddenly, instead of viewing my mother as someone who didn't give me what I needed growing up, for the first time I could clearly see her as a fellow human being, not that different from me—a person who had suffered tremendously as a child. I recognized that she was just as starved for affection as I was. A flood of love and compassion for her filled my heart to near bursting.

We never said "I love you" in our home growing up, but saying "I hate you" was as easy as saying "Good morning." The words "I love you" were too terrifying—a sign of weakness, vulnerability, and a mushy brain. In fact, I don't remember ever hearing that phrase growing up except at the movies.

I was determined to break that taboo. I was going to say "I love you" to my mother, even if I choked on the words.

The following afternoon, I watched as my mother sat down at the kitchen table with the familiar red-and-white checkered tablecloth, right next to the window looking out at the garden. She had just poured herself a cup of tea and was about to read the newspaper. I sat down across from her. A wave of love washed over me.

I took a deep breath and exhaled slowly. "Mummy, I'd like to tell you something. I'm so sorry for being such a difficult child and for being so mean to you and saying angry things, like calling you a 'mean witch' and giving you a hard time. I am so grateful for all you've done for us and all the sacrifices you made for your children."

My mother looked puzzled, as though she didn't comprehend my words. After a few seconds, her face softened. "You weren't such a bad girl. You were actually very sweet."

I was shocked by what she said. Was this the same mother who told me earlier in my life that I belonged in a mental hospital and that she couldn't believe she gave birth to a monster like me? The same mother who had slapped and hit me dozens of times? I quizzed her to see if she could remember anything bad that I had done or said to her when I was young. It was as though she had suddenly developed selective amnesia.

My mother's brain instantaneously rewired itself right in front of me, dropping all memory of the pain that I had inflicted on her with my angry words. She couldn't remember any of it. I had no idea brains could change that quickly.

I summoned my courage and reached over and took my mother's hands in mine. I forced myself to look into her green eyes. Making sustained eye contact was not something that had ever come easily to me, probably due to low self-esteem. With my heart racing, I managed to say, "I love you, Mummy." I had never been so frightened in all my young life. I closed my eyes and held my breath, waiting for lightning to strike me dead.

When I opened my eyes, I saw the tears running down my mother's face. She put her head down onto her folded arms and cried. At that moment, I realized that I had never seen my mother cry.

The tears rolled down my cheeks as my heart opened, fully aware of the magnitude of the scene in front of me. I knew that something profound had just happened, something that would permanently alter my life—for the better.

I understood for the first time that the act of *giving* love can be just as fulfilling as *getting* love. Giving my mother unconditional love empowered me and filled my bottomless pit at last. Gone were the insatiable longings for her love and approval.

To this day, my kitchen table is covered with an old-fashioned red-and-white checkered tablecloth to remind me of the transformative moment with my mother that changed my life.

My mother began calling me every week and writing me long, handwritten letters. We became close friends and freely expressed our support and encouragement of each other. At the end of each phone call, I forced myself to say, "I love you, Ma," and then quickly hung up the phone. Eventually, with repetition, the words flowed from my mouth more naturally. After many months went by, my mother began responding to my parting words by saying, in a constricted voice, "I love you too, Rickie."

Chapter 15

WRAPPING UP

WITH DR. SAMUELS' GUIDANCE, I took an unblinking look at myself and decided that I needed to make some changes.

I thought about how I wanted to move through the world and what I would need to do to become the person I aspired to be. I earnestly intended to recreate myself.

I made a list of the traits that I admired in various people, both in people I knew and people I had read about, and then I practiced becoming that composite person. At first I felt like I was acting a role on the stage, pretending to be someone else. Eventually, with persistent practice, I felt I truly embodied the composite persona I had created. Of course there were times, usually under duress, when I slipped back to my old mode of reacting—especially when around my family.

To begin my new life, I decided I needed to sincerely apologize for any wrongdoing by the "old" me, whether intentional or unintentional. I wrote carefully thought-out letters to the family members with whom I'd had conflicts and on whom I'd inflicted my share of pain. In the letters, I outlined my crimes as I saw them: relentlessly teasing and taunting my older brother, George, until he would chase me around the dining room table and into the yard; ridiculing and hitting John; and shaming and criticizing Susie because I was jealous of her intellect and her ease with boys.

I asked for their forgiveness—but got no response. In fact, to this day, no one remembers getting those letters. But the nature of my relationships with those siblings changed noticeably. At last, we were kinder to each other.

I continued to monitor my behavior to make sure I was not causing harm to anyone—and when I did something that I recognized was unkind, I admitted my wrongdoing and asked for forgiveness. It felt liberating to take responsibility for my actions and emotions and to let go of feeling like a victim and blaming others for my problems.

Many years later in medical school, when I learned about Alcoholics Anonymous and its 12 steps to recovery program, I realized I had tapped into some universal insights about becoming a conscious, awake human being through my work with Dr. Samuels.

During my last year of college, my mother telephoned me and asked if she could come for a visit. Neither of my parents had ever visited me in college. When she arrived, she was distraught in a way I'd never seen before. She had turned to me because she didn't know where else to go. She was of the old school and didn't believe in "hanging dirty laundry out for the neighbors to see."

She revealed to me that my father wanted to divorce her. He was having an affair with a woman from the college where he served as the dean of students. My mother, terrified of being on her own at this late stage of her life, asked me for guidance. "What will I do, Rickie? How will I support myself? Where will I live? I'll be all alone."

I felt helpless in the face of my mother's anguish. I had never seen her allow herself to be so vulnerable. She let me hold her in my arms and stroke her head, something I had never done before. My heart ached for her. I told her I would talk to my father. I was sure he would change his mind.

In the end, my father did change his mind, thanks to the strong opinions expressed by his daughters. My parents stayed together until my mother died 15 years later. The last few years of her life with my father were a time of deep healing, love, and tenderness—something they had both longed for throughout their marriage.

Shortly before my last semester of college, suspecting that Jeff and I would part ways at some point, I came to the sobering realization that my degree in art would not likely help me earn a living. If I had to live off the sale of my art, I would surely starve to death.

At the last minute I switched my major to education and crammed into the one remaining semester all the courses that I would need to meet the requirements to graduate with a teaching certificate.

As the time of graduation approached, my therapy sessions began to wind down. When I thanked Dr. Samuels for his help, he said I was his favorite patient. I didn't think psychiatrists were supposed to say things like that to their patients. He went on to say that I was remarkably healthy both mentally and emotionally—a far cry from the "mixed up" young woman he had treated at the start of therapy, "with an inaccurate and seriously distorted view of herself."

"All your longings as a child and young adult to understand life and be a good person have paid off and given you the fire to sort through what it all means. Now you have the tools and insights—that map and compass you were searching for—to navigate your life and reach your destination, even through the inevitable bad times. You are the captain of your ship. No more trying to fit someone else's template for who you should be. Your life is unique and won't resemble anyone else's life.

"You must embrace who you really are, Erica. Just as your father told you as a girl, you can indeed choose who you want to be and what you want to do with your life. You will find your purpose. Just be true to yourself and it will happen. Look at me—I was among the first Black psychiatrists to study in Zurich. I dared to dream big. And you can too. You're ready to discover your own path and fully claim your authentic life. I am so proud of you, Erica."

The tears spilled down my face as he spoke. I could see that his eyes were moist as well.

I will always be deeply grateful for the role Dr. Samuels played in helping me find my way. His brief and easily deflected forays into inappropriate behavior during our sessions did not diminish my gratitude.

His parting words to me were, "I hope you will stay in touch with me—not as a patient. I want you to write to me and let me know how your life unfolds."

I did indeed stay in touch with Dr. Samuels. Every few months I wrote him letters, which he responded to. Six years later, on my way home from South America, I stopped by his clinic to say hello and thank him in person for helping me find my way in life.

The secretary asked for my name and then said to go into his office and have a seat. He would be in shortly. When I walked into his office, I was shocked to see a familiar picture that hung on the wall behind his desk. It was a giant enlargement of a little Instamatic photo that I had included in one of the letters I sent him a few years after graduating from Antioch. The photo was of me on horseback, herding sheep at dawn on the Navajo Reservation.

> *Hmm. I wonder how his patients feel that he has a large photo on his wall of a former patient. Something about it doesn't feel right to me.*

As I stood wondering why he had hung the photo of me on his wall,

Dr. Samuels walked into the office with a big smile on his face. He gave me a strong, lingering embrace and then sat down behind his desk. He said he was on his lunch break and had some free time to talk with me.

When I asked about the photo, he said he wanted a reminder of the human potential for finding authenticity and meaning in life. He wanted my story to inspire others.

After I left, we continued to remain in touch sporadically. When he shared with me his fantasy of divorcing his wife and marrying me, I stopped writing to him for fear of encouraging that thought. But in spite of how our friendship ended, I will always be grateful to Dr. Samuels for helping me in my quest for understanding myself and understanding others.

It would be accurate to say that Dr. Samuels helped launch me onto my path in life. Once I had discovered my authentic self, I imagined the journey ahead of me as bursting with possibilities.

In May of 1970, when our college classes ended, Jeff and I did not attend our graduation ceremony. Our eyes and hearts were focused elsewhere, pulling at the bit to experience life on our own terms. We went in opposite directions that summer, each following the path that called out to us. Our stated plan was to reunite at the end of the summer, although we both knew that our marriage would probably not last. A year later, we officially divorced.

Switzerland was my immediate destination for the summer. I wanted to visit my relatives and get to know my Uncle Ernst better, my mother's younger brother, a most unusual Swiss medical doctor.

Chapter 16

UNCLE ERNST

Summer 1970

DURING MY CHILDHOOD, Uncle Ernst had been the subject of heated controversy in my family. My mother claimed he was a genius. My father claimed he was a quack.

I was determined to learn more about my uncle and what he did. I wanted to resolve the genius-or-quack question for good.

Uncle Ernst had invited me to stay a month with him in his home where his clinic was located. I assumed I would follow him around the clinic like an investigative journalist, interviewing him and learning about his work. I stuffed plenty of pens and a few spiral-bound notebooks into my backpack for that purpose.

When my train arrived at the station in the town of Landquart, I saw Uncle Ernst standing on the platform to meet me. He still looked the way I remembered him from the time we lived in Germany—a tanned, slender man of medium height with thick, wavy brown hair; an owlish face with intense greenish-blue eyes; and thin lips that were barely visible. In his mid-fifties, he appeared stiff and reserved, as though he lacked exposure to the world outside of medicine. His English was formal and stilted, reminiscent of the style found in literature of the nineteenth century. I wanted to give him a hug but restrained myself, not wanting to cause him discomfort.

On our walk from the station to his home, after a long stretch of awkward silence, he abruptly said, "Your fast will begin today." I didn't understand what he meant.

I stopped walking and looked at him with bewilderment. "What fast?"

"You will be on a fasting cure for a fortnight, followed by another fortnight of slowly introducing food back into your diet. The food will be all raw." He continued walking.

> *What is a fasting cure?*

Completely puzzled by his words, I switched to French, thinking that maybe in French he would be able to explain what he meant more clearly. He said the same thing in French, but instead of saying that I would not be eating any food for a fortnight, he said it would be two weeks. Two weeks somehow sounded worse than a fortnight.

"You mean I won't be eating anything for two weeks? Won't I die from starvation?"

> *I'm too young to die. I'm only 21. My life is just beginning. This sounds crazy.*

He answered, "You will be able to drink water. You will not die. You might get weak."

"But Uncle Ernst, why do I need to fast for two weeks?"

His answer took me by surprise. "Because you are American. You are toxic."

"Toxic?" That sounded like a harsh word usually reserved for something nasty in the environment, like an oil spill. "But Uncle Ernst, I'm strong and healthy."

"Americans eat unhealthy foods and eat and breathe chemicals. The fasting cure will clean you out."

I had a sinking feeling that I had made a bad decision to visit Uncle Ernst. He was surely a quack. My father was right. The idea of no food for two weeks was not appealing; in fact, it sounded scary.

> *I'm probably going to starve to death. If I survive, I can only eat food that hasn't been cooked? I've got to figure out a way to escape this place and go home—and just admit that I made a mistake in coming to see Uncle Ernst.*

While I was trying to hatch an escape plan, we arrived at a large stone building. Uncle Ernst showed me around the clinic located on the first floor of his home, and then walked me to my room upstairs. If I had any questions, I could ask Helen, his assistant.

I looked around my small, monastic room. I saw two tall glasses and several large pitchers of water on the nightstand. A pile of books written in English, French, and German had been carefully stacked on the table in the corner of the room. I flipped through several of the books and noted that the topics all related to natural methods of healing, including the benefits of fasting and eating an all-raw, organically grown diet. They also addressed the effectiveness of medicinal herbs, Oriental medicine, sauna therapy, wheatgrass, coffee enemas, and walking barefoot on the earth. In the bathroom, I noticed an enema bag with a long, snake-like tube for flushing out the intestines. It looked sinister.

I lay down on the firm, narrow bed and wondered how long I could endure a fast. To distract myself, I began to read one of the books.

The content grabbed my attention and gave me the feeling that maybe there was, after all, some legitimacy to his bizarre practices. After a few hours of reading, a sense of excitement and curiosity captured me. I decided to postpone my escape for a few days and see what would unfold.

Helen knocked softly and entered my room to greet me. She was friendly but seemed quite nervous, like someone who is fragile and easily upset. She asked if I had any questions.

I asked her how she first met my uncle. Helen said that "Herr Doktor Bauer" had saved her from the "insane asylum," as they called it in those days.

Helen and her older sister, Agnes, had schizophrenia. Agnes had been hospitalized off and on for years, while Helen resisted hospitalization. When she heard about Herr Doktor Bauer's remarkable abilities to cure some mental illnesses without medication, she made an appointment with him. She was 29 at the time. Uncle Ernst put her on a strictly raw, whole foods diet. Within days she no longer had the signs and symptoms of schizophrenia.

Many years later, I realized that Helen's seemingly miraculous cure could be attributed to the raw food diet she ate, a diet that excluded all grains. No grains meant that she ate no gluten. I knew from my own medical practice that for some people who are genetically susceptible, the gluten protein has the potential to affect the functioning of the brain and contribute to "brain fog" and mental illness, along with a host of other maladies.

Helen had gradually worked her way up the ladder in the household, beginning as a devoted patient who volunteered her services at the clinic as an expression of gratitude. Over time, she became Uncle Ernst's medical assistant, receptionist, secretary, and all-around personal assistant. Ultimately, decades later, she became his wife when she was 72 and Ernst was 89. Both made the leap into marriage for the first time.

In these new surroundings and facing this strange order to fast, I felt lonely and disoriented. Although I found Helen a bit odd, I didn't want her to leave. I asked her a stream of questions. She filled me in on some of Ernst's history and how he had discovered this different way of treating disease—or rather, curing disease.

Ernst had completed his medical training in Zurich and began his professional life as a conventional doctor, practicing what he called "schoolbook medicine." When World War II broke out, he served as a doctor in the Swiss army.

Toward the end of the war, Ernst became increasingly weak and emaciated. His weight dropped to 90 pounds and his skin turned yellow. A palpable tumor grew on his liver. He was convinced the cancer was from the mold that contaminated the food rations during the war, especially the bread.

Many years later, during my training in environmental medicine, I learned that certain strains of mold that grow on bread and other foods produce toxic chemicals that have the potential to cause various illnesses, including liver cancer.

Helen said that Ernst went to see many specialists. No one could help him. Finally a doctor referred him to a famous homeopath in Geneva, Dr. Pierre Schmidt. Uncle Ernst arrived in Geneva in critical condition. With the alternative treatments that his doctor prescribed, including fasting, enemas, raw food, and homeopathy, the tumor began to shrink and eventually disappeared over the following year. Ernst regained both his strength and his weight. He felt better than he ever had in his life.

While growing up, Ernst was struck by the fact that his father's medical patients kept coming back, in need of more treatments. He concluded that his father's conventional doctoring methods were not curing his patients. By contrast, Dr. Schmidt's chronically ill patients did not need to come back for more treatments. Many of them were cured outright. This observation strengthened Ernst's resolve to leave conventional medicine behind and devote himself to learning and practicing the methods of natural healing.

Once Ernst had earned a reputation as an accomplished doctor of alternative medicine, he was dismissed from the drug-oriented Swiss medical society. Thirty years later, after famous people across Europe sought out his care, the Swiss medical society formally invited him back. He politely declined. He had no interest in enhancing his status. His mission in life involved helping his patients feel better.

Helen took me on a little tour of the home and clinic. In the waiting room, about a dozen patients were speaking various European languages, but I also heard Russian and the Queen's English. I asked Helen to wait while I briefly talked with some of the patients. They spoke in tones of reverence when referring to Herr Doktor Bauer, recounting all he had done to cure their "incurable conditions" and letting me know the extent of their gratitude.

Maybe my mother's assessment of her brother was right.

If everything that his patients said about him was true, then maybe Uncle Ernst really was a genius—way ahead of his time. Perhaps my father called him a quack simply because he didn't understand the kind of alternative medicine that Uncle Ernst practiced.

Helen took me to the clinic, where gadgets and equipment partially filled the treatment area, along with a sauna, a device for spinning blood, and hundreds of vials of homeopathic remedies. A wide wooden balcony served as the place for sun therapy, lined with several chaise lounges. Helen said Uncle Ernst advised his patients to get a little sun every day and to walk barefoot on the earth as part of their get-well program. In those days, the general public considered such advice pretty nutty. Now, almost 50 years later, it's considered progressive thinking with some science to back it up.

After our little tour of the clinic, I started to feel a gnawing hunger I could no longer deny.

"Helen, I can't stand the hunger. What would happen if I snuck something to eat?"

Helen smiled and said, "Ah—your uncle will know, because every morning when he makes the rounds of his patients, he asks them to stick out their tongues. He can tell immediately if someone has cheated by the color of the tongue."

"Really?" I was disappointed.

"You must drink many glasses of water. It will help you feel better. It's best if you lie down and rest right now." After she left my room, I looked through more of the books on natural healing, then turned out the light.

My sleep was filled with dreams of food. In one of the more vivid dreams, I climbed out the window, ran into town in my nightgown, and knocked on the door of a restaurant. I ordered a bratwurst on rye bread with mustard. It tasted divine. After filling my stomach, I ran back, climbed through the window, and crawled into bed.

I awoke in a panic thinking that my nocturnal escapade had really happened and that Ernst was going to know from looking at my tongue. In the bathroom, I stuck out my tongue to see in the mirror if it had changed color. It still looked the same. I could relax.

The second and third days of the fast were difficult. I felt weak and hungry and did not enjoy myself at all.

How am I ever going to complete this fast? I have eleven more days to go. Oh my God. This is Hell.

I drank glass after glass of the mountain spring water from the pitchers on the nightstand to fill up my stomach and get a few minutes of relief from the gnawing ache. A mild headache came and went throughout the first few days. My sweat and urine smelled acrid and my breath smelled like something rotting in a garbage can. I looked at my tongue in the mirror. It was coated with a white film. The skin on my face and throughout my body had little red bumps that looked like tiny pimples.

Maybe this is what Uncle Ernst meant when he said I was toxic. Maybe the toxins are coming out now.

I liked the image of my body cleaning itself out. I bathed two or three times a day in hot water and watched the sweat run down my body after I got out of the tub. Once a day I walked down the hall and sat inside the wooden sauna for a half hour and did more sweating.

After a couple of days, I got over my revulsion and resistance to giving myself the daily enemas. Eventually I went willingly into the bathroom to do the dirty deed, holding onto the vision that my insides were becoming sparkling clean. When I wasn't bathing, drinking water, looking at my changing body in the mirror, taking saunas, or doing enemas, I lay on my bed in a daze, dozing off and on, too weak to socialize or read with any kind of concentration. I wrote nothing in my diary.

Uncle Ernst made his daily morning appearances to check on me. I had gotten used to his nervous awkwardness when he interacted with people—including with me, his niece. Sometimes he spoke in German to me, sometimes in French or English.

As he stepped into the room, he would inquire how I was feeling. No matter what my answer was, he said, "Ah. That's very good. Very good. Yes," followed by a nervous laugh. As predicted, he had me stick out my tongue to assess my status and then he checked my pulses in the Chinese style of diagnosing. He said that I had "kidney deficiency." I had hundreds of questions to ask him, but each time I began to question him, he told me to read the books and learn from them. Later he would talk to me. I wasn't sure when "later" was supposed to be.

On the fourth day of fasting, something magical happened. I awoke feeling refreshed, rested, clear-headed, and actually bubbling with energy—mental and physical energy—while at the same time experiencing a deep and pervasive sense of peace. My hunger had mysteriously disappeared. I had no discomfort anywhere in my body. Colors looked brighter; the air smelled pure and intoxicating. I felt alive in a way that was new to me. Strange and wondrous feelings filled my mind and body.

Everything in my life and in the world felt perfect just the way it was, no matter what. There was nothing to fix—not even the heinous things in life, like the Vietnam War that hung in the back of my mind.

Streams of love coursed through my being. It was a different kind of love, impersonal and unconditional, a love for everything, everybody, every living and nonliving thing. No boundaries separated them from me. The sky outside, the water in the pitcher on the nightstand, the tree on the other side of my window, the mountains on the horizon, the chair next to the desk—I was all of them and they were me.

Tears of love and gratitude for life flowed down my cheeks as my hands rose spontaneously to my heart, one over the other. My chest felt like it would burst right open from intense feelings of love.

With these expanded feelings came a sense that I knew everything that had occurred in the world in the past and that I already knew the future. There was nothing I didn't know, because the past and future merged within me in the present moment. With certainty I knew the contents of everyone's mind and heart, even strangers.

> *This must be what it feels like to be God. How can I ever admit I had feelings of being like God? Is it sacrilegious? Will people think I'm psychotic? Do I ever dare tell anyone what happened?*

Fortunately, I easily let go of my logical, skeptical brain and resisted the temptation to talk myself out of what I was experiencing so vividly, even if it lay beyond reason.

In college I'd heard people talk about these kinds of blissful "oneness" experiences, but at the time, the altered states they described were mere concepts to me—nothing I had ever experienced. Their altered states were drug-induced. Mine were starvation-induced, probably related to certain chemicals produced in the starving body.

I lay on my bed for hours, mesmerized as if I were watching a gripping movie. What I experienced was more real to me than "real life." I got my very first glimpse into the world of the spirit, beyond the veil that separates us.

I spent the whole rest of the day in an altered state, a parallel universe that I never wanted to leave. At some point, it dawned on me that if I didn't record the experience in my diary, I would never believe this experience had actually happened. And the memory of it would surely fade over time. I would think I had imagined everything that occurred.

And how is anyone going to believe me when I tell them what happened?

When I read my diary entry years later, my words sounded ecstatic and incoherent. But the entry clearly conveyed that I was in the middle of what would become a profoundly life-changing, mind- and heart-expanding experience.

The morning of the fifth day, I awoke to a continued but less intense state of expanded and altered perception, without hunger or discomfort. My energy was moderately good. When Uncle Ernst came by to check on me, I gave him a slightly censored thumbnail sketch of what had unfolded, too embarrassed to reveal the whole extent of the wondrous inner events for fear of sounding crazy.

Ernst looked at my tongue and felt my pulses. "Aha. Very good. Yes. Very good. Hmm. It's time for you to go outside and walk in the mountains. I will make arrangements for you to walk with another patient." He bowed slightly forward in a gesture of respect and gave me a little lipless smile with a sparkle in his greenish-blue eyes. Then he left the room to continue on his daily rounds at the nearby hotel within walking distance. The hotel lodged Dr. Bauer's patients exclusively. The overflow of out-of-town patients found lodging in private homes where their medical needs could be accommodated.

Shortly after Ernst's visit, Helen knocked on the door and said that a young French woman, Marie Madeleine, would be waiting for me downstairs in an hour to go hiking in the Alps together. Helen gave me a jar of water and a little rucksack to take up the mountain.

How am I possibly going to be able to hike up a mountain after not eating for five days? Willpower and determination only go so far.

Marie Madeleine was beautiful, with dark hair and olive skin and clear, shiny green eyes. She was slightly older than me, devoutly Catholic, and from a rural area of France. She spoke only rudimentary English, so we kept our conversation in French. She told me that my uncle had helped her get well from a supposedly incurable disease, a disfiguring and oozing rash that covered much of her body. When she experienced a relapse years later, she returned to Switzerland to do the fasting cure and raw foods diet for a second time. We had both been fasting for five days.

I expressed to Marie Madeleine my concern that I would not be able to hike up a mountain in my current state. She reassured me that the place we were going would not require much hiking. We would take an aerial tram up the mountain and then walk along a mountain path to an alpine lake.

It was a beautiful, pristine sunny day. I was still in a mildly expanded state of consciousness. I continued to feel unconditional love for all beings. Riding in the tram up the mountain, I had the sense that I understood what was in the minds and hearts of each of the passengers. I knew their past and I knew their future—not all the details, just a general sense of knowing.

Am I delusional? Is what I'm feeling real? It sure feels real.

Marie Madeleine and I walked slowly, in silence, for about a half hour along a vertiginous mountain path, lined with low-growing pink heather. We came to a breathtaking alpine meadow full of mountain flowers blooming with all their hearts in joyful splashes of color. A few of the flowers I recognized, like mountain arnica and calendula with their yellow, daisy-like appearance, the cobalt blue gentians, the purple thyme draping itself over the rocks, and the iconic white edelweiss. The fields of flowers stretched in all directions. The scene was so exquisitely beautiful that it was almost painful.

> *I wonder if a person could get a heart attack from being overjoyed. What if my heart literally explodes from being so happy? The papers would report, "American girl found dead in the Alps. The cause of death determined to be an overdose of happiness."*

We slowly meandered along the narrow path through the flowers until we came to a tiny alpine lake, our destination. It was mid-afternoon and warm. Without hesitation, Marie Madeleine took off every single piece of her clothing as I looked on with curiosity. She lay on the ground completely naked, seemingly oblivious to the possibility that a hiker might see her. I lay on the ground a few feet from her with my clothes on. Ten minutes later, my clothes came off too. We both lay on our backs spread-eagled, looking up at the sky in reverent silence. I wanted to stay forever. When the sun dipped to the horizon, we reluctantly dressed and headed back to catch the last tram going down the mountain.

On the sixth day, I awoke with the same sense of wellbeing, without hunger or discomfort—but my energy level had dropped. When Uncle Ernst came by on his morning rounds, I told him about my excursion in the mountains and expressed an interest in going again while I still had some energy. He invited me to join him on his weekend hike in the mountains the next day. I eagerly accepted.

I spent most of that day reading from the books that Ernst had left for me in my room. Intense thirst for information about this strange new world I had entered kept me focused on the material, although I frequently needed to doze off between chapters.

The seventh day fell on a Sunday. I awoke feeling good, but without the intense high I had experienced over the previous three days. When Uncle Ernst fetched me for our hike, he was wearing knickerbockers and knee socks, and he carried a rucksack and walking stick.

After a short train ride, we boarded a bus that took us partway up the mountain to the trailhead. The scenery was spectacular.

I wondered if I'd be able to keep up with Uncle Ernst. I was strong, but I hadn't eaten anything in a week.

> *Well, Uncle Ernst is 56 years old and I'm 21. So, maybe I can keep up since he's an old man.*

We hiked along a path, following the contour of a meadow that cut across the slope of a tall mountain. It was exhilarating to be so close to the tops of the snow-covered peaks. Within a few minutes of hiking, I was out of breath and lightheaded and had to sit down. Ernst was patient with me and told me to walk more slowly, in a measured way, placing one foot in front of the other, keeping up a steady but slow pace. I was too winded to even attempt to fill the welcomed silence with talk.

Eventually we stopped for "lunch," which meant that I drank two quarts of water while Ernst slowly ate a handful of nuts, one by one. I watched closely, tracking each nut as it entered Ernst's mouth. Within an instant, saliva filled my mouth. It was the first time in a few days that I'd felt hunger. The gnawing sensation in my stomach returned as the gastric juices started to flow again.

> *How can Ernst live on such a small amount of food? How does he have the willpower to stay on this kind of a diet? How does he have so much energy? Where does it come from? Doesn't he miss all the delicious things that normal people eat?*

As the day progressed, I needed more frequent and longer rest stops, no matter how slowly I walked. During the rest stops, Ernst started talking to me in more depth. He spoke in his usual voice, barely louder than a whisper, punctuated by his nervous laugh. He seemed almost pathologically shy, as if it was an effort to be around people.

I asked Ernst why he had decided to go into medicine. Did he do it just because his father—the grandfather I never knew—had been a doctor? He said no, he had made his own choice for his own reasons. He spoke about his painfully cruel and abusive childhood, which I knew about from my mother's stories of the same harsh treatment. Ernst gave some heartrending examples of what it was like to grow up after his beloved mother died when he was two years old.

For Christmas one year, when Ernst was four years old, his stepmother gave him a wooden rocking horse that he didn't want. She beat him because he didn't show appreciation or thank her on his own, spontaneously.

Around that same time, his stepmother locked him out of the house as punishment; for what, Ernst could no longer remember. Neighbors who came to visit found little Ernst on the back steps, shivering in the snow, with only his shorts and a shirt on.

> *No wonder Ernst is so awkward around people and ill at ease. And shy. He's been brutalized. And no wonder he's not married and has no close relationships with anyone beyond his devoted and grateful patients. He's married to his medical practice. I bet he's never had sex in his life.*

I asked Ernst if he was bitter and angry with his stepmother for brutalizing him and my mother. And did he feel hurt that his father didn't protect his children from the abuse? His father was working long hours in his clinic and absent from his children's day-to-day life.

Ernst said no, he had no anger. He had forgiven everyone who hurt him and was grateful, because it was precisely the pain from his childhood that made him want to help others who were suffering.

He chose medicine as a means to fulfill this desire, having grown up with his father's clinic downstairs in his childhood home.

> *How can he forgive something so terrible? And be grateful for it? How exactly did he convert that torture into wanting to help others? This is like something from the Bible, something Jesus would do. I think I'm in the presence of a very great and humble man. And I'm his niece. I'm so lucky. I hope he'll let me be his student.*

Ernst said that if I'd like to join him the following weekend for another excursion, it would be a pleasure for him. I agreed with enthusiasm. After I returned to my room, I realized the outing would fall on the last day of my fast. I doubted I would be able to participate in anything at that point due to weakness.

On days eight through twelve I felt significantly less energetic, verging on extreme weakness and lethargy, but without hunger. My morale was good. By the twelfth day, I had lost around 18 pounds even though my weight at the beginning of the fast was normal for my height. I loved feeling exceptionally lean, without a trace of fat. At least once a day in my room I slowly ran my hands over my whole body and enjoyed the way it felt. The image reflecting back to me from the mirror looked quite different from the Antioch College graduate who had showed up at the train station 12 days before.

That girl had headaches, mood swings, energy swings, episodes of congestion without any obvious explanation, low-grade anxiety, and bloating and swelling after certain meals. And she was sometimes way too serious. This girl in the mirror was not only lean and tan—she was relaxed and looked happy and peaceful and loved to laugh and smile. You could see in the mirror's reflection a light shining from the inside.

Uncle Ernst

Must be that all those enemas and saunas have made me sparkling clean on the inside. Maybe I was toxic after all.

I was tired of staying in my room and reading. Helen suggested that I go to the hotel and talk to some of Ernst's patients. She said that I would learn a lot about Ernst and his treatments just by listening to their stories.

The hotel staff had been trained to make raw meals according to Uncle Ernst's specifications. The patients said the meals were delicious. I couldn't wait to try out this new way of eating. But while I was still fasting, I made sure not to show up at mealtimes. That would have been too tempting.

Now I could finally fulfill my fantasy of being an investigative journalist during my stay in Switzerland. Since Ernst was painfully introverted and unavailable most of the time, I would interview his patients as the next best thing.

Helen had told the patients I would be coming. In the sitting room with notebook and pen in hand, I looked for a friendly face. A woman beamed a broad smile at me from across the room. She must have guessed I was Doktor Bauer's niece from America. Her name was Hilda.

She has that same light shining out of her face that I saw in the mirror. She must have cleaned herself out to get that light.

Hilda was from Germany and spoke a little English, so we switched back and forth from English to German. Hilda had intestinal cancer. She had tried *Schulmedizin*, or school medicine—the European way of saying "conventional medicine"—including surgery and chemotherapy. But the tumors had come back and spread throughout her body. Her doctors said that her prognosis was poor and that she needed to get her affairs in order. But she wasn't ready to die; there were things she wanted to do with her life.

Hilda heard about Doktor Bauer and his reputation for helping people with terminal diseases. He said she would need to fast for 21 days, given the gravity of her condition. She became extremely weak and emaciated during the three weeks and spent most of her time sleeping in bed when she wasn't giving herself the requisite enemas.

At the time of our interview, Hilda had been eating raw food for two and a half weeks. She said she felt better than she ever had in her entire life. I wanted to hear more about what Uncle Ernst did with her in terms of treatment, but by this time I was so exhausted and weak that I had to slowly walk back to my room and lie down.

The following day, I went back to see Hilda and finish my interview with her. She said that Doktor Bauer had given her regular acupuncture treatments during her fast, along with something called *Blut Waschung*, in which he drew a pint of blood from her veins, then ran it through a machine that exposed the blood to ozone and to ultraviolet light, a procedure for disinfecting the blood of viruses.

Doktor Bauer also told her to lie in the sun for a half-hour every day and walk barefoot on the grass or in the dirt at every opportunity. In those days in Switzerland, no one used pesticides or herbicides, so it was safe to walk barefoot.

Ernst lent Hilda many books to read from his vast library, as he had done with me, including books about how what we eat can affect our health for better or for worse.

After a couple hours into our second interview, I had to go back to my room and lie down. I was losing stamina each day. Hilda ended the interview by saying that she thought Doktor Bauer had saved her life and I was lucky to be his niece. She hoped I would return one day and work in the clinic with him as a fellow doctor. I smiled. The idea of becoming a doctor seemed fanciful and outside the realm of what I was capable of. I was not a genius like Uncle Ernst.

Day 13, the penultimate day of the fast, arrived on a weekend. Uncle Ernst had invited me to spend the day with him ice skating in Arosa, a well-known ski resort in the Alps where he eventually moved his home and clinic a few years after my visit.

> *How am I going to be able to ice skate? I haven't eaten even one crumb of food for 13 days.*

The train to Arosa passed through lush green valleys and along a little mountain river. Uncle Ernst performed his strange exercises in the aisle of the train, such as deep knee bends with his back straight as a rod, which years later I realized were related to the Alexander Technique. He had been prescribed the exercises to improve his posture and open his constricted chest. I felt ill at ease watching my uncle's uninhibited behavior cause stares and neck craning of nearly every passenger in that section of the train. I felt relieved when we reached our destination.

The ice rink was large, in the open air, with a close-up view of the Alps in the background. Ernst rented skates for me. I could hardly believe I could skate after nearly a fortnight of fasting.

On the ice, I felt so weak that I had to move in slow motion and stop frequently to rest and catch my breath. I skated in little bursts of energy, from one side of the rink to another, and then I hung onto the railing at the edge until I recuperated enough to make another crossing on the ice. Meanwhile, Uncle Ernst seemed to be thoroughly enjoying himself in his own world, twirling around and making figure eights and skating backwards. I envied him and wished I could join the fun, but weakness overtook me.

After about an hour, I had no more energy left for skating. I sat on a chaise lounge with a view of the mountains while sipping my two quarts of water for lunch. Eventually Ernst joined me. We sat in silence as he ever so slowly ate the lunch of apple, pear, and nut paste that Helen had prepared for him.

I remembered how concerned I was initially that I wouldn't be able to survive without food for a fortnight. I was glad I hadn't carried out my plan to escape. I would have missed one of the most incredible experiences of my life. Seeds had been planted in my mind and spirit—seeds that would one day get watered and germinate, radically altering my path in life.

I spent much of the last day of my fast lying on the ground by the river, listening to the sound of the water flowing over the rocks, watching the sky, smelling the mountain air, and feeling the sun warm my slightly chilled body. I thought about my friends and family and wondered how I could possibly relay to them what had happened on this mind-blowing, life-altering trip to see Uncle Ernst.

Thoughts of the following day, the day I would break the fast, flitted through my mind, but mostly I stayed in the present moment. I experienced no hunger, as though my entire digestive system had shut down.

∼

The day for re-introduction of food finally arrived. Helen had told me that my first and only meal for the day would be a banana. She said I must reintroduce food in tiny amounts to avoid upsetting my digestion, since it had been shut down for a fortnight.

At midday, Helen brought me one-third of an organic, overripe, black-skinned banana on a large white plate, along with a wooden spoon and a cloth napkin. She briefly spoke to me, reminding me to eat slowly, and then left the room, allowing me to experience in solitude the ecstasy of eating again.

I peeled the two-inch chunk of banana ever so slowly and ritualistically. The light yellow blob looked soft and mushy. It smelled inviting, exotic. I took a piece of the banana and licked it once, then again. I closed my eyes to focus on the rush of sugar into my body. I had never tasted anything sweeter.

After about an hour, I finished licking the little chunk of banana and scraped off every trace of banana from the peel. My better judgment kept me from eating the remains of the peel.

My senses had become keen during the fast—so keen that I could smell the sweet banana scent in the air the rest of the day as I lay in bed reliving my eating experience and wondering what the next day would be like. Weakness, still present, left me limp.

On the second day of eating, Helen gave me one-half of an overripe banana. The third day, I got an entire black-skinned banana. On the fourth day, one of Uncle Ernst's patients invited me to pick cherries in his orchard.

A ladder leaned against an old cherry tree. I climbed up and started picking the fruit. Helen recommended that I eat only 20 cherries that day so I wouldn't get diarrhea. I carefully counted out the cherries as though they were pieces of gold. I pressed each dark red, ripe cherry against the roof of my mouth with my tongue and let the nectar drip down my throat, drop by drop. Fortunately, no one was around to hear the irrepressible moaning sounds of ecstasy.

By the fifth day, my diet had expanded significantly to three or four portions of fruit. I began to feel energetic and ready to become part of the world beyond my room. The time had come to join the other patients at the hotel for the artfully prepared, all-raw and organic cuisine. A smorgasbord filled the serving table, including nuts, nut milks, and nut pastes; fresh vegetable juices; whipped avocados with lemon and tomatoes; salads made with greens, grated beets, carrots, and turnips, topped with sprouts; and crackers made from mashed and dehydrated seeds.

Before being with Uncle Ernst, I found raw vegan food like this pretty unappealing and unsubstantial. Now, everything I sampled—no matter how ordinary—tasted like food for the gods. My taste buds had become exquisitely sensitive after the prolonged detoxification.

My energy returned and, along with it, a sense of adventure. I wanted to learn more about what Uncle Ernst did, exactly. I asked for permission to shadow him for the last ten days of my month-long visit. He agreed. Following his schedule became my next challenge.

He rose at five in the morning, did his odd exercises, then called patients for homeopathic consults from seven to nine o'clock. Next came a little breakfast that typically consisted of homemade nut butter and vegetable juice.

After breakfast, Uncle Ernst attended to his patients in the clinic the entire day until the evening, stopping only briefly to eat a handful of nuts around lunchtime. Sometimes he worked until nine in the evening. I couldn't keep up with him and had to excuse myself by the late afternoon to rest.

Ernst respectfully asked each patient's permission to let me observe the interviews. The patients seemed very willing, and some were even enthusiastic to have Doktor Bauer's niece present in the room to observe. Maybe they thought I was a medical student.

Ernst treated anyone who came to see him, including local immigrant workers who had no money to pay him. He even tried to learn his patients' native languages so he could speak to them in their mother tongues and help them feel more at ease. Ernst was too modest to tell me how many languages he spoke fluently, but I heard him speak at least six or eight different languages while interviewing patients from other countries.

Along with impoverished patients, Ernst also treated the wealthy and those who were in the news. One of his patients told me that several cardinals from the Vatican traveled regularly to see Ernst and that he even treated Queen Elizabeth's mother while she was visiting Switzerland. The royal court doctor practiced homeopathy and was a colleague of Uncle Ernst. Konrad Adenauer, post-war chancellor of Germany, came for treatment in the early 1960s. But, of course, I never would have learned this information from Ernst himself.

Ernst constantly learned new healing modalities. Two or three times a year, he attended conferences abroad to learn cutting-edge techniques. A few years before my fasting cure, he had studied acupuncture in France with a famous practitioner.

Uncle Ernst taught me that underneath all the various healing modalities lies the real foundation of health: our lifestyle, including what we eat, drink, and breathe; the thoughts we focus on; and the quality of time we spend in nature.

Although Ernst did not converse with me much except when we were hiking, he did stress to me above all else the importance of food in making people sick and making them healthy. He explained that one reason why I felt so good on the fast was that I had some serious food allergies that were affecting my health.

I have food allergies? Really? I don't notice them.

He must have read my mind. He said that most people don't know they have food allergies because they eat the foods that they're allergic to every day and have become used to feeling bad. They rarely associate their symptoms, such as arthritis, fatigue, and frequent colds, with the foods they eat.

Ernst invited me to join him every time he went hiking. On those hikes he began to seem more relaxed with me. He expressed interest in learning about my life, what it was like growing up in my family, and what his sister was like as a mother. In turn, he shared with me more about his life and philosophy. He confided in me that he felt bad about not marrying Helen. He had written a letter to my mother asking her for advice. My mother said that he needed to marry Helen and turn her into "an honest woman."

Ernst said that he forced himself to consider marriage, but at the last minute called it off because he realized he couldn't fulfill his "duties as a husband."

>*What were those duties?*

I translated his statement to mean that he was thoroughly married to medicine and had nothing left to give to Helen. They ended up getting married 30 years after that conversation in the mountains. Uncle Ernst was in his mid-eighties.

I was an eager student, hungry for all the information that Ernst and his patients offered to me. I didn't want the month to be over. I asked Ernst if I could stay on as his apprentice. He said, "Not now. You're not ready."

>*Not ready? What in the world does he mean by that? I bet he thinks I'm not smart enough.*

I didn't feel comfortable asking for an explanation, but I tossed around lots of possibilities in my mind. I would come to understand—two decades later—what he meant. He wanted me to grow up and learn about life and about medicine before I apprenticed with him. When I was a practicing medical doctor, he invited me to return to his clinic as his apprentice for a few weeks.

The day I left Uncle Ernst's home and clinic in Switzerland, I had a powerful intuition that the month I spent with him would bear fruit someday and would eventually change the course of my life. I wasn't sure how or when that would happen.

At the train station, we said goodbye. There were few words spoken beyond my expressions of gratitude. Although reason told me not to be too exuberant, I couldn't help myself. I threw my arms around my uncle and kissed his cheek. His body stiffly received my gesture. As I stepped back, I saw a big smile illuminating his face.

Uncle Ernst continued to see patients until he was 91 years old. We stayed in touch through letters and visits over the next 37 years—until he died at 93 from complications that occurred after falling and fracturing his hip.

Chapter 17

PEACE CORPS

THANKS TO THE TWO YEARS of insightful and eye-opening talk therapy with Dr. Samuels, by the time I graduated from college, I had slayed the demons, dragons, and goblins of my youth—the self-doubt, the false beliefs about myself, and the fear of not being good enough. I became acquainted with my authentic self and couldn't wait to embark on my search for purpose.

With a degree in education and a teaching certificate in hand, I began looking through the trade journals in search of interesting teaching positions. Only one out of over a hundred job openings attracted my attention. The Bureau of Indian Affairs had an opening for a fourth grade teacher at a boarding school on the Navajo Reservation in a remote area of northern Arizona. Without clearly understanding why, I applied for the position. I knew I had to trust my inner compass even if I could not explain to enquiring friends and family the logic behind my choice.

I went to the reservation without knowing anything about my students or their culture. After several cross-cultural blunders, misunderstandings, and inability to communicate with the students, I was beset by loneliness and despair. I thought about leaving and going home.

My Navajo teacher's aide saw how much I wanted to connect with the students and how frustrated I was. She offered to teach me about

Navajo culture and traditions in order to help me understand my students. After seeing my eagerness to learn, she taught me a few words of Navajo, considered one of the most difficult languages in the world.

Once I started learning to speak in Navajo, the children began to trust me. They responded to my interest in them with an intense desire to learn English so they could tell me about their lives. During the first year of teaching, it was exhilarating watching the students go from barely speaking English to seeing some of them win a regional speech contest.

Once I was able to cross the cultural divide, a strong bond developed between the students and me. They welcomed me into their homes and extended families and invited me to participate in their sacred ceremonies. They introduced me to their enchanting land and the richness of their ancient traditions. I participated in a world that few non-native people have ever experienced.

As I was drawn ever deeper into their culture, I witnessed a series of profound events that included miraculous healings, peyote ceremonies, and encounters with ancient spirits. Most chilling of all was surviving a face-to-face encounter with a mountain lion, which a Navajo elder later explained was my spirit guide. That same elder predicted that I would one day bring powerful medicine to the people.

Many years after leaving the reservation, I returned to serve the Navajo people as a medical doctor. I recounted the full story in my first memoir, *Medicine and Miracles in the High Desert: My Life Among the Navajo People.*

From those transformative years living among the Navajo people, I learned how much I enjoy teaching—but not the simple act of conveying information. The teaching needed to be meaningful and empowering, and in an atmosphere of empathy and genuine caring.

I developed a thirst for learning more about people and places that were different from what I was familiar with. Although I had been raised as a child among several different cultures due to my father's work, as an adult I became most drawn to Native people.

While I was in high school, one of my sisters worked for a couple of years at the Peace Corps headquarters in Washington, DC. Listening to her recount the stories told by returning Peace Corps volunteers so intrigued me, I fantasized about signing up as a volunteer someday.

After I left the Navajo Reservation, I decided it was the perfect time to join the Peace Corps and learn more about Indigenous people in other parts of the world. I signed up at the end of 1973 when I was 25 years old.

I requested a position working in the Andes Mountains of South America with Quechua-speaking people whose ancestors belonged to the Inca Empire. The Peace Corps assigned me to Ecuador for my two years of service. The experience turned out to be far different from what I could ever have imagined.

The Peace Corps had arranged for the volunteers to have three months of language training in Ecuador's capital, Quito, before we dispersed to work in our assigned locations.

During our training, we stayed with families who spoke no English. Since I had already learned to speak Spanish during the semester when Jeff and I lived in San Miguel de Allende in Mexico, I could focus more of my attention on learning about the land and the people of Ecuador, their customs and culture.

When not in class, I roamed around the magnificent city of Quito, admiring the colonial architecture in the center of town, a blend of European and Indigenous styles. Quito sits high in the Andean foothills at over 9,000 feet. A 15,696-foot active volcano called "Pichincha" looms over the western side of the city.

One morning, as I walked around the city, the clouds overhead began to part, giving me a jaw-dropping glimpse of a gigantic, snow-covered, perfectly cone-shaped mountain in the distance to the south. I stared breathlessly at the celestial apparition in front of me while my heart raced with excitement.

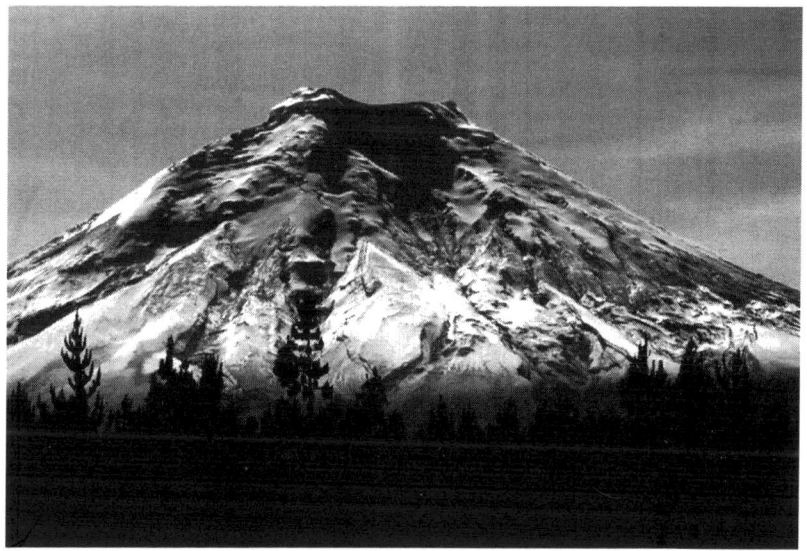

Cotopaxi is the highest active volcano in the world, at 19,347 feet.

A man on the street, seeing this gringa in a state of unabashed wonder, said to me in Spanish, "Señorita, what you are looking at is Cotopaxi. It is part of a chain of 27 volcanoes we have in Ecuador."

At that moment a wave of intense desire to climb those massive volcanoes washed over me—even though the idea was wild and unrealistic and seemed to come out of nowhere.

Before the man could walk away, I asked, "Señor, if someone wanted to climb the volcanoes, what would they need to do?"

FROM MOUNTAINS TO MEDICINE

He answered, "Only experienced mountaineers climb these mountains because they can be dangerous." He said I could get more information at the National Polytechnic Institute, which sponsored a well-known climbing group called "El Club de Andinismo Politécnico."

Full of anticipation, I walked all the way across town to the Polytechnic Institute, the Ecuadorian version of MIT.

The woman receptionist told me that the climbing club was mostly for male students of the Institute. I said I just wanted to sit in on a meeting and listen to what they discussed. She gave me the time and date of the next meeting.

My host family urged me not to even think about climbing the volcanoes because of my lack of experience and the risk of getting killed. On top of that, I was a woman and shouldn't be thinking about those sorts of things, they said.

I showed up to the meeting of the Club de Andinismo right on time. The room was full of men; I didn't spot a single woman at that meeting. One of the men approached and asked if he could help me. On impulse, I said I wanted to join the climbing club. The man looked at me with disbelief, but eventually took me seriously when he saw how determined I was to join.

He asked me if I had any experience climbing mountains. I assured him that I had climbed quite a few mountains in the United States, including Mt. Washington, Mt. Jefferson, and Mt. Adams in the Presidential Range, part of the White Mountains in New England.

Fortunately the young man had never heard of the mountains I listed and did not ask me their height. If he had, he would have discovered that the tallest of the three I listed, Mt. Washington, was only 6,288 feet, a mere anthill compared to the nearly 20,000-foot volcanoes of Ecuador.

In describing my ascents in Spanish, I had unwittingly used the words "hiking" and "climbing" synonymously, which misled the man into thinking I was an experienced technical climber. This miscommunication on my part later led to some awkward and embarrassing moments.

The student said they were planning to climb Cotopaxi the following weekend and that I could come along. I told him I didn't have any gear with me other than my sturdy hiking boots, warm clothes, and the basic camping gear I had brought from the States. He said the club had extra gear I could borrow.

The student conferred with the other members of the club. They all agreed that, before I joined them on the trip to Cotopaxi, they needed to take me to a local climbing area to see how well I climbed and what gear I needed. That Saturday, we drove to a snowfield to practice walking with crampons on the glaciers. It wasn't long before I had to confess to the men that I didn't know how to use a rope, tie knots, use an ice axe, or even put on crampons, much less walk with them on.

The men looked surprised, understandably. They walked a few yards away from me and talked among themselves. I waited, holding my breath, knowing that I could be in big trouble for having unintentionally misled them into believing that I had prior technical experience climbing big mountains.

A steady stream of irrational thoughts flooded my brain. I had visions of the men abandoning me in the wilderness as punishment for misleading them. Surely I would freeze to death on the snowfield—or a hungry jaguar that smelled my flesh from the edge of the jungle many miles away could come and eat me alive. The embassy would have to call my parents and tell them the sad news about their daughter's death. I felt stricken with remorse thinking that I could cause my parents such terrible anguish and grief.

After what seemed like a very long time, but was maybe only ten minutes, one of the young men walked over to me and said that he would teach me everything I needed to know about snow and ice climbing in the Andes. His name was Jorge. He gave me a friendly smile. Awash with relief and gratitude, I heartily shook his hand. The tension left my body and my shallow breathing deepened.

I couldn't help wondering why this young man elected himself to help me. In any case, I felt very fortunate.

Jorge was about my height and looked extremely fit, with a strong, slim body and a smiling face with shiny brown eyes. Although Jorge was younger than me by five years and still in college, he became my mentor in the mountains. Unlike the other men who were more reserved, Jorge wasn't shy around me. He made sure I put on the crampons correctly and tightened the straps. He taught me how to tie the various knots to secure myself with the rope and asked me to repeat the process until I had the knots memorized. He showed me how to dig the ice axe into the hardened snow to negotiate steep and icy inclines.

By the time our practice session ended, my brain felt inundated with new information, especially regarding the different knots.

The time arrived to put what I'd learned from Jorge to the test on our ascent of Cotopaxi. I rode with nine men from the climbing club in a van that took us to the base of Cotopaxi. It was a two-hour trip on the Pan American Highway, the road that begins in Alaska and ends at the tip of Argentina. Jorge and I sat beside each other in the back seat.

No te preocupes, Erica. Todo saldrá bien. Te cuidaré en la montaña. He reassured me that everything would be fine; he would look after me on the mountain. Jorge's words calmed my smoldering fears and kindled a feeling of warmth and gratitude toward him—my new friend and mountain mentor.

We drove to a flat area at the base of Cotopaxi and got out of the van. I had to tilt my head back to take in the volcano, staggered by its immense size.

As we donned our gear, Jorge made sure I had everything I needed. I noticed that much of the men's equipment was homemade, including their gaiters, crampons, jackets, some of their backpacks, and even their ice axes. Many of the men had brought blankets, not having the luxury of a sleeping bag. I felt spoiled that I had a down jacket, a down sleeping bag, and a high-quality backpack with a large frame. I had some enviable gear—but no experience.

In those days, before accelerating climate change, the glacier extended all the way down to about 12,000 feet, where we began our ascent. We climbed up to the wooden, box-like shelter, called Refugio José Ribas, with our packs full of climbing gear, sleeping gear, and food. Each of our packs probably weighed between 40 and 50 pounds. I arrived breathless and light-headed, having traveled from approximately 9,000 feet in Quito to the shelter at 15,958 feet, a 7,000-foot elevation gain in one day. The men appeared well acclimatized, without evidence of rapid breathing or excessive fatigue.

On the way to the shelter, the young men spoke animatedly about the trip and their lives in general. They asked me a stream of questions, curious to hear about my life in the United States, the Peace Corps, and why I chose to come to Ecuador. My answers were short. I tried not to let them see how much I struggled to catch my breath and how exhausted I felt during the few hours it took us to ascend the lower part of the glacier and reach the shelter.

We happened to be the only climbers on the mountain, so we had the little shelter to ourselves. After we prepared a simple dinner with soup and hot drinks in the late afternoon, the group leader told me I should get some rest because we would leave the shelter around midnight. We needed to take advantage of the cold nighttime temperature, which would allow our crampons to grip the ice and packed snow while the surface remained hard. After the sun rises in the sky, the snow gets slushy on these equatorial glaciers.

Anticipation kept me from sleeping. My heart pounded in my chest at a much faster rate than normal. I could feel a high-altitude headache coming on. I took two aspirin, praying I wouldn't get the dreaded altitude sickness that the men had warned me about. They described its characteristic symptoms—fierce headaches, vomiting, dizziness, weakness, and mental confusion. The leader encouraged me to stay hydrated.

We melted the snow in a camping stove and filled our canteens with water. I drank so much water that I had to go to the outhouse and pee almost every hour. The frequent peeing was caused not only by the heavy intake of water, but also by nerves; I worried that I wouldn't be able to make it to the top with these highly acclimatized men.

The shelter had no heat, leaving the inside near freezing. I wondered how the men would stay warm with just their thin blankets to cover them and without down jackets.

At around seven o'clock in the evening, I crawled into my frigid sleeping bag and shivered, eventually drifting in and out of a restless sleep. At some point in the night, Jorge lay down next to me. Within minutes I could hear his deep, rhythmical breathing. I wished I could fall asleep that quickly.

At midnight, Jorge roused me from my half-awake state and told me to gear up and get ready to leave. I had gone to bed with my clothes on, including my wool hat, so I only had to put on my climbing boots and gaiters.

After sharing a pot of coffee, we left the shelter at half past midnight. We roped up and headed up the steep mountain. It was an icy cold, clear starry night, thankfully without wind. Jorge asked me to hook my carabiner onto his rope, about five feet behind him. A third climber roped in behind me. Without a headlamp, I followed Jorge closely, trying to step exactly into his tracks as we made our way up the switchbacks.

In the shelter, the men had warned me about the crevasses that we would traverse on the glacier and how careful we had to be so as not to fall into one of them. The first crevasse we came to had a wide opening. I look down into the bottomless chasm and shivered with fear.

Jorge said we had to step up our pace so we could beat the sunrise. He urged me to set a slow but steady pace, which would allow me to go farther between rest stops.

I had to overcome my concern about slowing down the group and allow myself to do what I needed to keep going, which meant stopping and panting after each step while bending over and leaning on my ice axe for support. Since I only stopped for a few seconds each time, I didn't think I was breaking Jorge's no-stopping-to-rest dictum.

Halfway up the mountain the terrain became steep and treacherous. I felt like I was walking sideways up an extremely narrow staircase. The left foot crossed over in front of the right foot, then the right foot slowly moved past the left foot on the uphill side, carefully keeping the crampons' spikes from catching on our gaiters and throwing us off balance. I briefly contemplated the possibly fatal consequence if I lost my balance. Having to focus so intensely on each step kept me from becoming paralyzed with the fear of falling to my certain death.

At six o'clock in the morning the sun appeared, filling the horizon with a spectacular red and orange glow. The sunlight gave a boost to everyone's morale. The view took my breath away—any breath I still had. From where I stood, I had a clear view of the chain of volcanoes, including Chimborazo, the highest volcano in Ecuador at over 20,000 feet. I wished I had the energy to fully appreciate the magnificence of the skyline.

I regretted that I'd forgotten to bring my little Instamatic camera. I consoled myself with the promise that I would be back to climb this mountain more than this one time—after I got acclimatized to the altitude in Ecuador.

Every time I thought we were almost at the top, Jorge let me know it was a false summit. The altitude at the true summit is 19,347 feet. We arrived there at seven o'clock, after six and a half hours of climbing. I was too exhausted to register anything except a desire to lie down in the snow.

After exchanging congratulatory hugs and handshakes with each of my climbing companions, I unclipped the carabiner that connected me to the climbing rope and collapsed onto the snowy ground. My headache had become explosive, and I felt light-headed.

Someone in the group let us know that the temperature was 6 degrees below zero Centigrade. My mind was too wiped out to estimate how that number would translate to Fahrenheit. I only knew that my body shivered from the freezing cold.

After a few minutes of catching my breath while staring off into space with an empty mind, I made myself rise and walk around the enormous crater. I wondered if anyone had ever fallen into the crater. The strong smell of sulfur kept me from getting too close.

Our leader said that we had to rope up and head down before the sun melted the top layer of snow. We drank from our canteens and ate our snacks, then headed down the mountain a little after eight o'clock.

My legs felt like rubber. I could barely hold myself upright. I slipped and fell frequently but was able to arrest myself with my ice axe as Jorge had taught me. I tried not to think about what would happen if I slid all the way down the mountain—or fell into a crevasse and was never found. A wave of sadness washed over me as I thought again of the grief my parents would feel if they lost their daughter and had no way to retrieve her body. I silently asked the gods of the mountain to give me the strength to make it down the mountain safely. With all the determination I could find within me, I made it to the shelter. When I stepped inside, I saw a wooden bench and promptly lay down on my back and stared up at the beams on the ceiling as my mind churned out a stream of existential questions.

Why is climbing this mountain so important to me? Why am I willing to take such big risks to reach the top of the mountain? What does climbing have to do with finding my life's purpose?

After we all rested for about a half hour, we ate our lunch, drank the last of the water in our canteens, and then continued our journey down the mountain. Jorge taught me how to *glissade*, a climbing term that means sliding down the mountain. I sat on the snow with my legs outstretched, imagining myself in a toboggan. I flew down the last part of the glacier, with ice axe positioned, ready to jam it into the snow in case I got too out of control.

We finally reached the end of the glacier and stepped onto *terra firma*. We stashed our gear in our backpacks and headed back to Quito in the van. We rode the whole trip back mostly in silence, tired and lost in our own thoughts. The mountaineering experience left me feeling a strong bond with my new friends.

The bond I felt made me think about men coming back from war. I wondered if they felt something similar, having made it through harrowing experiences, relying heavily on each other's support. I felt an especially strong bond with Jorge, who had taken me under his wing and offered me his expert guidance.

When we arrived back in Quito, giddy with the joy of being alive, I shook the hand of each of my new friends and expressed my gratitude for being included on the climb and for all the encouragement they gave me on the ascent. I wanted to give each of them a big, warm hug—but I didn't dare, not knowing the customs of Ecuador regarding male-female interactions.

When I shook Jorge's hand, he grinned and said, *Felicitaciones, Erica. Aprendes muy rápido. Espero volver a verte pronto. Cuídate.* "Congratulations, Erica. You learn very quickly. I hope I see you again soon. Take good care of yourself."

Back in Quito, I felt like I had been to Mars and back. It was difficult to fully convey to my compatriots in the Peace Corps what had happened on the mountain. I'd experienced a rarefied world high in the sky that few people knew about in those days.

I called my parents and spoke to them briefly about the climb. My father expressed vicarious excitement. My mother worried that I could have gotten hurt, even though I left out some of the more scary details.

The three-month Peace Corps training program for the volunteers came to an end. Soon I would be leaving Quito and traveling north to start the first of two work projects the Peace Corps had assigned to me. Thoughts of the mountains and my new mountaineering companions never left my mind.

Chapter 18

HOME GARDENS

FORTUITOUSLY, THE PEACE CORPS had somewhat arbitrarily assigned me to teach topics related to health, first aid, nutrition, and home gardening in rural communities—even though I had never received formal training in any of those fields.

Without realizing it at the time, I repeatedly chose paths that would contribute something vital in preparing me and bringing me ever closer to finding and fulfilling the purpose of my life, which remained to be determined. Whatever that purpose turned out to be, I knew it needed to include teaching people something that could make a positive difference in their lives.

On my application, when asked about my interests, my list extended to the bottom of the page. Near the top I had yoga, meditation, running, hiking, gardening, biology, and nutrition. At the end of the list, I wrote, "In summary, I'm interested in Life."

At the Ecuadorian government's request, the Peace Corps assigned me to a town called Guayllabamba, located about 40 kilometers north of Quito, where I would teach the people how to create home gardens for growing vegetables to supplement their limited food choices and improve their nutrition.

Instead of keeping a diary, I wrote long, detailed letters to my parents by candlelight each night. Upon hearing about my assignment, my father sent me packets of seeds to use in my model home garden.

An official from the town suggested I use a plot of land near the *acequia*, the community's irrigation ditch. He assigned two men to prepare the soil for planting and building a little fence around my plot to keep the animals out. The men seemed surprised when I enthusiastically pitched in with the manual labor.

The pumpkin seeds my father sent sprouted and grew profusely, obviously suited to the climate and soil. The other seeds that sprouted included Swiss chard, broccoli, garlic, onions, corn, peppers, cucumber, potatoes, mustard, radishes, beets, lettuce, cabbage, and tomatoes—a veritable sea of vegetables.

The friendly townspeople came by to look at my garden and marvel at the large variety of vegetables, but they did not express much interest in growing their own food.

One man said in Spanish, "Why should we grow food when we have the money to go to the store and buy canned food?" When I encouraged them to eat quinoa due to its protein-rich, health-enhancing qualities, another man said in disgust, "Quinoa is for *Indios* and other poor people."

All the people in Guayllabamba looked like Indians or Mestizos to me. I got the impression that considering yourself to be Indian wasn't so much about your family heritage or the color of your skin—but about the amount of land, money, and education you had.

In Guayllabamba I lived rent-free in a tiny room in an adobe house I shared with the landlady. Although she treated me with kindness and curiosity, she was one of the many people who told me firmly, "Only *Indios* eat quinoa. You are wasting your time teaching the people in our town to grow their own food."

Geez! What do I do now?

Awake at odd hours of the night, I would mull over how to respond to the impasse I faced. Sometimes I had to pee in the middle of the night. I didn't want to stumble through the dark all the way to the outhouse, located quite a few yards behind the house. So I peed in a jar that I kept under my bed. In the early morning, I walked out to the front porch and poured the jar of urine onto the ground below. The dilute urine had no smell, so I didn't worry about being inconsiderate of others. After a few weeks, some scraggly-looking little weeds surrounding the stone steps leading up to the porch turned into enormous, colorful quinoa plants and little poinsettia trees. The landlady exclaimed in amazement, "*Dios mio!* I've never seen the plants grow so fast and look so healthy! You bring *magia Americana* to our country." I held my breath, trying not to laugh at the idea of "American magic."

Most weekends I walked into the town's center, filled my hand-woven shoulder bag with exotic fruit like *cherimoyas*, and then hopped onto an overcrowded bus headed to Quito. The colorful bus looked like it would tip over from the piles of goods and caged animals headed to market, strapped precariously onto the roof. I almost never found a seat and had to stand with the others, all pressed together.

In the city, I met up with my mountaineering friends to climb yet another of the countless massive volcanoes in the surrounding area. After spending an exhilarating weekend with them high in the Andes, I felt waves of loneliness wash over me as I returned to Guayllabamba on Sunday evening.

In exasperation over the home gardening fiasco, I finally traveled to Quito to speak with administrators in the Peace Corps and Ministry of Agriculture. They understood the futility of trying to convince the people of Guayllabamba to grow their own vegetables to improve their diets. They reassigned me to a similar home gardening project in an Indigenous community a bus ride away from Guayllabamba.

While I continued to sleep in my room in Guayllabamba, I commuted every weekday to the Indigenous community. After only a week of adjusting to my new setting, I began looking forward to each day working with the people. They had no biases against growing their traditional foods and learning about how to grow more vegetables, so they eagerly responded to my teaching efforts—unlike the people in Guayllabamba. A recurrent phrase I heard in broken Spanish was *Que Dios le pague*, "May God repay you."

My father mailed me another box stuffed with packets of vegetable seeds, which I added to the seeds provided by the Ministry of Agriculture. I showed school-age children how to plant the seeds and grow vegetable gardens on the grounds next to their school. I talked with their parents about the importance of good nutrition, including the benefits of eating vegetables.

The children and their mothers clustered around me whenever I spoke with them. Although shy, they showed rapt interest in the information I conveyed. A man stood nearby to translate my Spanish into Quechua whenever necessary.

The boys wore pants and ponchos, while the girls wore white blouses, shawls, and dark skirts held up by colorful woven waistbands. None of the children wore shoes. Their broad feet gave the appearance of stability and direct connection with the earth. As I looked at them, with their wide smiles and their shiny, copper-colored faces framed by jet-black hair, my heart filled with warmth and affection.

The children quickly learned how to grow vegetables. They used a portion of what they harvested to add to their school lunches and brought the remainder to their homes. When a family had more food than they needed, they generously shared the excess with other families.

The children eventually passed on what they had learned and taught the rest of their community members how to create their own vegetable gardens. The vegetables supplemented the grains and potatoes they grew in their fields.

I noticed how much I enjoyed teaching—especially teaching a topic like nutrition that could significantly improve people's lives. With the villagers now growing their own vegetables in their home gardens, it was possible for me to teach them about nutrition.

The Indigenous people received care packages from the churches overseas. The care packages from the States usually contained soy and corn flour, and powdered milk. The mothers mixed all the ingredients together, creating a pancake-like concoction that they cooked over a fire outside near the school so that the children could eat these culinary curiosities along with the scraps of food they brought from home.

The children ate their food sitting on the ground. When it rained, they either didn't eat at all or they ate and got wet. Seeing them eat in these conditions touched me. The list I kept in my little notebook included figuring out how to get money to build a kitchen and dining room adjacent to the school.

I told my connections at the Ministry of Agriculture that the children lived too far away to walk home for lunch. The officials approved of the projects I described and offered their financial support.

With the funding I procured, the people would have the means to build the community kitchen and dining room I had envisioned for the school. Once the headman of the village gave his permission to proceed, the men in the community began working from dawn to dusk on the project. From inside the school, the kids and I could hear a cacophony of hammering. Within just a few weeks, they managed to complete the two adjoining structures.

On opening day in the brand-new community kitchen, the girls made lunch for all the students, the two local teachers, and me. A celebratory mood filled the air. Most of the people, young and old, were smiling with exuberant pride in the new structures they had built.

With the remaining funds, the community built an outdoor, wood-burning oven made of adobe so that the mothers could gather weekly to make bread. The Indigenous people enjoyed working communally. Although they had only their hard labor to offer, they offered it with unquestioning commitment to the projects we embarked upon.

Enthusiastic about my work, Ministry of Agriculture officials invited me, all expenses paid, to spend a week in the city of Loja in southern Ecuador so I could observe the model nutrition education program the city had implemented.

I thought it would be fun to invite Jorge, my climbing companion, to travel with me to Loja. We had become close friends. I noticed how much I had begun to miss him when we were apart.

We took the train, which ran on the highest train tracks in the world—according to Jorge—and enjoyed a spectacular ride. We found lodging with a couple of Peace Corps volunteers in the area who befriended us. I discovered that the nutrition program in Loja was pretty similar to what I was already doing in the Indigenous community. The week passed quickly.

The trip to Loja deepened the friendship between Jorge and me. We went climbing with the club on many weekends. Sometimes we simply stayed in Quito and wandered around the beautiful city by ourselves.

Jorge excelled in his studies and didn't need to spend much time studying on the weekends. In fact, I had the impression that all the students in the climbing club were highly intelligent and would eventually be moving on to outstanding careers.

I sensed that Jorge was becoming increasingly more interested in me by a certain mischievous look on his face. I realized that I was starting to have romantic feelings for him as well. When he reached out to hold my hand for the first time, my face flushed and a wave of heat ran through my body. I could feel our hands become sweaty. We both acted as though nothing was happening between us.

Jorge invited me to visit his family in Quevedo, a town in the hot and humid coastal region of Ecuador. His entire family enthusiastically greeted me—parents, five sisters, and three brothers. They treated me with warmth and endearing hospitality—and endless questions. They made sure I was well fed and well taken care of, including making sure that I had plenty of mosquito netting over my bed when I slept so I wouldn't get malaria. I thoroughly enjoyed being part of their family for the weekend.

One time while we were leisurely exploring Quito, Jorge put his hand on my shoulder, looked into my eyes, and said impulsively, *Vamos a algún sitio.* (Let's go someplace.) He had a great big naughty-boy grin on his face.

Hmm. I wonder where that someplace is.

After Jorge took me to visit his family, I realized that he viewed me as his girlfriend. I suspected what he meant was, "Let's go to a hotel and make love." And that's precisely what we whole-heartedly did.

Although I did not ask him directly, I had a feeling that I was Jorge's very first girlfriend. He was an eager student, and I was an eager teacher. I tried my best to give him an unforgettable introduction to the fine art of lovemaking.

In the process of this hands-on mode of teaching, I couldn't resist falling head over heels in love with him. Before we left the hotel, we swore eternal love for each other.

Immediately after we made the oath, I wondered how I could possibly keep my part of it, considering I would be in the Peace Corps for only two years and then I was planning to return home. Using purely wishful thinking, I reassured myself that everything would work out the way it was supposed to—and we'd find a way to stay together despite the daunting obstacles.

Chapter 19

ON THE RIDGE

During that first year in Ecuador, Jorge and I and the rest of our climbing group reached the summit of at least a dozen of the most spectacular volcanoes I could ever have imagined, including Chimborazo, the highest mountain in Ecuador at 20,700 feet.

It took me a couple months before I was thoroughly acclimatized and could keep up with the men, even while carrying a heavy pack. My days of desperate panting were over.

On one climb, when Jorge was with his family for the weekend, I went with a few of our *compañeros* from the climbing club to Antisana, a nearly 19,000-foot volcano located southeast of Quito, not far from Cotopaxi.

Antisana, the fourth-highest volcano in Ecuador, has three summits. The climb is extremely technical, requiring considerable experience with high-altitude snow and ice climbing, along with the appropriate equipment for vertical ascents up sheer ice walls.

On the drive to the volcano, we saw wild horses roaming the *páramo*, the vast, seemingly empty stretches of land that could be compared to the moors in England or the tundra in Alaska.

A few feet from where we parked our van, a condor stood with his enormous wings outspread imperiously. He stared at us with his beady eyes without moving his bald, pink head. His claws dug deep into a rabbit he had ripped open on the ground. Blood stained his beak. As we piled out of the van, the condor hopped a few times and then flew away, carrying the mutilated rabbit with him in his claws.

We set up camp high on the glacier, much higher than we usually set up camp. I could smell the sulfur fumes wafting down the mountain from the snow-covered crater just below the summit.

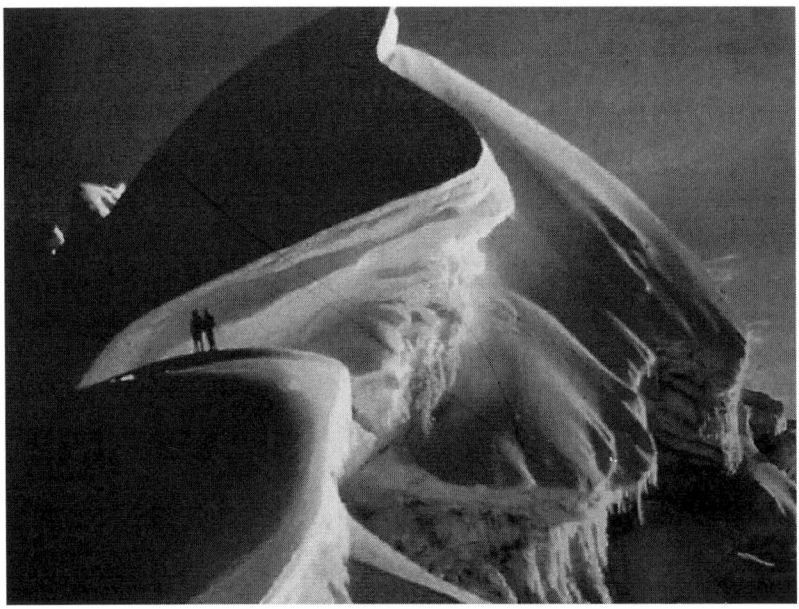

Antisana is the fourth-highest volcano in Ecuador.
The two climbers, members of the climbing club, are standing near the south summit of the pass on Antisana.
Credit for the photo goes to Santiago Rivadeneira.

When we rose at midnight to begin our ascent, I started coughing. I assumed the sulfur was irritating my lungs. As we trudged along, the coughing worsened, eventually accompanied by an altitude-related headache, a symptom all too familiar to me.

Just before we reached the first of the three summits, I realized that something was very wrong. I could no longer think clearly. I stumbled frequently and had become dangerously short of breath, with spasms of coughing.

I told the leader of our group that I thought I had pneumonia. Our leader, a Chilean professor at the Polytechnic Institute, of German heritage, had helped form the climbing club. The professor suggested I had *soroche*, or altitude sickness. He explained that I probably had pulmonary edema—meaning fluid in the lungs, which my mother had experienced when she and my father had come for a week-long visit.

The professor said that the low oxygen pressure at high altitude caused the blood vessels in the lungs to expand and leak fluid into the surrounding lung tissue, making it difficult to breathe. He suggested that I also had cerebral edema, for the same reasons, which explained why I couldn't think clearly or walk without stumbling.

Since Jorge was not on this climb, his best friend, Mateo, came forward and gallantly offered to escort me off the mountains. The professor said we needed to get off the mountain as soon as we could, but without endangering our lives.

I had met Mateo on other climbs. Reserved by nature, he remained genuinely humble and soft-spoken despite being obviously intelligent and highly competent in the mountains. In fact, Mateo and Jorge were considered to be Ecuador's best climbers. I had learned from one of my climbing companions that Mateo had heroically tried to rescue a team of climbers who died in an avalanche.

Mateo had always been courteous and kind toward me, lending a hand at any opportunity. As we rapidly descended the mountain, Mateo patiently answered my breathless, anxiety-tinged questions in his calm voice.

For most of the descent, Mateo kept me roped up on belay until we came to terrain that was less steep and less glaciated. I felt sure I had pneumonia and told Mateo I would need to somehow get to a hospital right away. Mateo responded, *No te preocupes, Eriquita. Todo saldrá bien,* reassuring me that everything would turn out well.

Then something quite strange happened. By the time we had descended to a much lower elevation, I stopped falling down and began to think more clearly. And then, even further down the mountain, the cough disappeared.

My symptoms were indeed from pulmonary and cerebral edema. I had just experienced my first episode of *soroche*. In the ensuing months I would be able to recognize altitude sickness in other non-acclimated climbers and help them get to safety.

Back on the flat land in Guayllabamba, I dreamed every night of the mountains, my mountain companions, and our adventures together. Although I thoroughly enjoyed my projects in the Indigenous community and found the work very meaningful, I nevertheless couldn't wait for the weekend to come so that I could get back into the mountains with my *compañeros*. My anticipatory excitement reminded me of the excitement I felt as a girl in anticipation of going on a hike with my father.

Over time, I began to see that climbing big mountains had meaning far beyond the simple act of climbing to the summit. The climbs served as a metaphor for my life and all the efforts I made at overcoming seemingly insurmountable obstacles—including self-doubts, feelings of not being good enough, and other self-limiting beliefs about myself.

An inner knowing convinced me that what I learned in the mountains would help me face the challenges yet to come—the kind of challenges that come simply from being alive and engaged.

Mountaineering taught me to persevere even when I was confronted with gripping fear and exhaustion. I saw that putting one foot in front of the other would eventually get me to the summit—even if the goal seemed impossibly out of reach. I came to realize that my body and mind had far more capacity to meet serious challenges than I ever could have imagined.

My mountaineering *compañeros* and I climbed as a tightly bonded team with a common goal. I learned to be part of that team, relying on my climbing partners for support and encouragement, and ready at all times to give the same in return. We made our way up the treacherous mountains together, we protected each other, we encouraged each other, and we celebrated with each other.

~

Jorge and Mateo wanted to climb one of the several peaks on a mountain called Sincholagua. That particular peak had never been summited before. It was one of the smaller peaks on Sincholagua, but it was treacherous.

Sincholagua is an eroded, extinct volcano. Its name comes from an Indigenous word meaning "steep upward," an appropriate name for this smaller but precipitous volcano.

When we reached the snow-covered, knife-edged ridge that would take us to the summit, Mateo and Jorge conferred among themselves. They concluded that the last stretch was too dangerous to climb because of the wind-blown and corniced snow hanging off the leeward side of the narrow ridge. If we took one misstep to the left onto the cornice, we would all fall over the edge to our death as the fragile overhang of ice and snow gave way. Now I understood why the peak had never been climbed.

Despite their warnings, I expressed a strong desire to try reaching the summit—even by myself if necessary. Jorge and Mateo discussed this possibility. Since there was no way to set an anchor in the snow to protect me or anyone else on belay for a distance much longer than the length of our rope, they suggested that we disconnect ourselves from the climbing rope and each climb unprotected. That way, if one of us fell, we would not pull the others with us to our certain death.

I knew I had to face this challenge, even if it meant risking death—not for the glory of being the first to climb this peak, but for other much more compelling reasons. Climbing this summit ridge symbolized to me the courage I would need in confronting challenges that lay ahead in my life.

During the time I lived on the Navajo Reservation, a mountain lion sniffed me a few inches from my face while I lay in my sleeping bag on a slab of red rock in southern Utah. After the terrifying encounter, a Navajo grandmother explained to me that the mountain lion was my spirit guide and had come to me to give me his "courage, strength, and intense focus," because I would need all of those for what lay ahead. She said I would face "many obstacles, some big and life-threatening." She went on to say that if I lived through them, I would have "a strong heart and powerful medicine to give to the people."

I wrote those words in my diary shortly after the grandmother spoke them, and then I forgot about them over the years. But I didn't forget what she said about the many obstacles that I would face: "some big and life-threatening." Those words helped give me the courage to keep going in the face of fear—and the strength to continue in the face of utter exhaustion when I didn't think I could take one more step. I had to strengthen my mind and body for whatever challenges lay ahead.

Seeking my purpose in life was like being on a mythological journey, full of demons and dragons and other terrifying monsters—but also full of wondrous sights and experiences, each teaching me something I would need to know on the way to reaching my destination.

Looking back, that terrifying ridge could have symbolized the scary goblins I had to get past on my journey forward. The goblins this time represented self-doubt and limiting beliefs about my capabilities.

As I walked along the knife-edged ridge, my mind remained intensely focused on each carefully placed step on the hard-packed snow. On the icy patches I could feel the spikes on my crampons holding my footing. My ice axe helped me maintain my equilibrium. I knew that one misstep would mean certain death. If I stepped too far to the right, I would tumble down a near-vertical slope. If I stepped too far to the left, I would be on the cornice, which could easily break off, leaving me flying through space. In the face of my intense focus and concentration, nothing existed beyond the present moment. My breathing became slow and measured, as though I was in a meditative trance.

When I reached the summit, a tiny pinnacle, I waited for the others. The scant standing space barely offered room for the other climbers. No one spoke. We immediately turned around and began our slow and painstaking trek back.

Once we got off the ridge, Jorge gave me a quick congratulatory hug and said he was proud of me. Mateo shook my hand and gave me a shy smile. We were jubilant to have reached a summit that had never before been climbed.

Coming down off the mountain, the irrepressible exhilaration and joy at being alive made me burst out singing at the top of my lungs. When we got to the bottom, we gave each other bear hugs and slaps on the back.

On the drive back to Quito, we sang songs. Jorge asked me to teach him one of the Beatles' songs that I had sung on our descent. I couldn't stop grinning and laughing at his charming accent while singing the English words to "Yesterday."

The climbing club subsequently christened the peak with my name, Pico Erica Elliott. I still have the clipping from the Quito newspaper about that climb and the naming of the peak. The laminated article hangs in my clinic, now yellowed with age.

One weekend when Jorge and I hung out in Quito together, he broke some painful news to me. He began by saying that the Hungarian government wanted the rights to some of the massive amounts of oil that had been discovered in the jungles of Ecuador. In exchange for those rights, the Hungarian government would offer full scholarships to high-achieving students to study at the university in Budapest. A few days before the weekend, Jorge had received a letter from the Hungarian government, offering him one of those scholarships to study engineering.

We both shed tears at the idea of being apart from each other. Jorge explained that getting a good education was essential for having a good life and was one of his highest priorities. But, without help, getting a top-notch education would have been unattainable due to the heavy financial burden on his parents.

Jorge asked me to go with him to Hungary. When I told him I couldn't renege on my two-year commitment to the Peace Corps, I could see the hurt in his face. He asked if I would wait for him and stay in touch while he was in Eastern Europe. I naïvely assured him I would, believing that I was capable of "waiting" for him—also known as being celibate—for three or four years.

Jorge's family asked me for a loan to pay for his airfare. I gave almost all the money I had brought with me from the States as a reserve fund in case of an emergency—a wad of dollar bills that amounted to $400. Jorge assured me that his family would repay the loan, which they did eventually—almost in full. I gave the loan willingly as a demonstration of my commitment to Jorge.

Since those days of making oaths of eternal fidelity, I've learned the harm that I can cause by making commitments that I cannot keep.

Chapter 20

FINDING MY PLACE HIGH IN THE ANDES

November 1974

AFTER I HAD WORKED FOR A YEAR in the lowlands, first briefly with the town of Guayllabamba and then the Indigenous community teaching health, nutrition, and home gardening, the Ecuadorian Ministry of Agriculture ran out of funding for further projects such as mine, due to a financial crisis that had swept the country. I would have to leave the community that I had come to love. The news left me sad and disappointed.

With time, my disappointment evolved into excitement about a new opportunity. I'd heard the Peace Corps officials mention the serious need for bilingual materials for teaching Spanish to Quechua-speaking Indigenous children who lived in isolated villages high in the Andes Mountains. I enthusiastically volunteered to take on this project. It seemed like a perfect fit, given my prior experience implementing bilingual and bicultural education in the Navajo boarding school where I taught for two years.

The people in Guayllabamba and the little Indigenous community had separate goodbye parties for me. In Guayllabamba, on the evening of my last day, a group of men gathered and played music while a few people danced drunkenly in the little plaza in the center of town. Store-bought food and alcohol appeared in abundance. At the end of the evening, the people lined up to shake my hand and say a few words of thanks.

In the Indigenous community, the men sang and played hauntingly beautiful Andean music into the night on homemade instruments, including drums, violins, flutes, panpipes, and a type of ten-stringed instrument called a *charango,* also known as an "Andean ukulele." The women and children made a veritable feast that included mounds of vegetables from the gardens. Some of the children presented me with homemade gifts, including a beautiful multi-colored shawl and warm socks. I had tears in my eyes as I hugged the people goodbye.

The Peace Corps arranged for me to take two weeks of Quechua language training in Quito. The instructor began by informing us that several words used in English originated from the Quechua language, words like *condor, llama, vicuña, guanaco, guano, coca, puma, quinine,* and *jerky.* Of course, the spelling of these words in Quechua looks and sounds a little different from the Anglicized versions.

After the language training, I lived for a week with a Quechua-speaking family to practice my new skills. The Peace Corps paid the family for providing me with food and lodging. I made every effort to avoid speaking Spanish during that week so that I could familiarize myself with the sounds of the Quechua language in everyday use. By the end of my immersion in language training, I had learned to use about 100 words in Quechua, enough to at least make rudimentary conversation.

Next, the Peace Corps gave me permission to choose the site where I would implement a pilot program in bilingual education. I wanted to find a place where the need was the greatest. The goal was to help the Quechua-speaking children learn Spanish so they could eventually get jobs in the city and support their destitute families. My role would be to develop the bilingual teaching materials.

I left Quito and hiked to a region high in the Andes where the people spoke very little Spanish. I walked from one hamlet to another. Most people fled when they saw the foreign woman wandering around, but a few brave people spoke to me warily in broken Spanish.

By the end of the day, I had chosen La Compañía de Jesús Cristo as I had heard that a bilingual Indigenous schoolteacher came weekly to teach the children Spanish in the old one-room schoolhouse. Although I hadn't met this teacher yet, I imagined she could help me implement my project of developing bilingual and bicultural teaching materials for use throughout remote areas high in the Andes.

The community, located on the lower slopes of the mountains at around 12,000 feet, was populated by impoverished families of *huasipungueros,* the indentured servants of the absentee landowners—a position just a few notches up from being slaves.

The region was beautiful, filled with seas of golden barley that made sensuous, undulating waves in the wind. Patches of quinoa plants of various colors added vibrancy to the cultivated slopes. The colors constantly changed hues as the clouds drifted by and the sun moved along its trajectory.

While checking out La Compañía, I thought it would be a good idea to introduce myself to the local priest, knowing that priests have a lot of influence, even in Indigenous communities. I found him sitting in the courtyard of his modest rectory, which stood next to an ancient, crumbling adobe church. He gestured for me to join him for a cup of tea. We spoke in Spanish. The old priest, dressed in his black cassock, had come from Spain in the 1930s to convert the Indians to Catholicism. He was the first white person to arrive in La Compañía. Within the first year he had learned to speak Quechua. Now he intended to retire and return home to Spain in a few days.

The priest spoke with a crisp politeness that barely concealed his overt suspicion of me. After a few minutes of small talk, he got to the point and grilled me about my motives for wanting to live with the Indians. He eventually understood that I was not a Communist and that I had no intention of starting a revolution.

The priest saw how earnest I was about wanting to live in La Compañía and help facilitate the children's education in Spanish. He gave me the contact information for the owner of a decrepit and partially collapsed hacienda at the edge of the hamlet where I might be able to live. The *hacendado* lived in Quito and only came to La Compañía once a month to pay his serfs their wages, the equivalent of 19 cents per day.

After much searching in Quito, I finally found the owner of the abandoned hacienda. He lived in a relatively luxurious compound in the foothills on the edge of town. He was middle-aged and slightly overweight, with an insincere smile. After we spoke about my situation, he reluctantly agreed to let me live rent-free in his decrepit building—on the condition that I would swear I would never try to "change the Indians' way of living or talk to them about religion." He made it all too clear that there would be trouble if I didn't fulfill my promise. He told me about a white anthropologist who had come to La Compañía in the 1960s. The people murdered him out of fear that he had come to harm them. As he said those words, I felt a fleeting wave of terror move through my body.

When the wife of the *hacendado* asked me if I was Catholic, I made the mistake of admitting that I was not. Clasping her hands together in a dramatic gesture, she said, "*Dios mio*, don't ever tell anybody. The Indians will surely kill you. They are very religious."

I managed to get out of that tight spot by claiming that I was an Orthodox Protestant, a religion that, I explained, was basically the same as Catholicism, only an American version. Fortunately, she believed me. After that encounter, I quickly trained myself to make the sign of the cross and, when appropriate, to give the benediction—in the name of the Father, the Son, and the Holy Ghost. I hoped I wouldn't end up in Hell as punishment for my survival tactics.

At the end of our conversation, the *hacendado* assured me, with a sardonic smile, that a *gringa* like me would not last long living in the primitive conditions found here. He predicted I wouldn't even last a week and suggested I get in touch with him after I let go of my "unrealistic illusions of living with *los Indios*." Giving me a flirtatious look, he said that he and I could go out one evening and have a drink together and he would tell me all about life in Ecuador. I had no intention of taking him up on that offer.

In late November of 1974, after making the necessary arrangements in Quito, I hiked back up the mountain with all my possessions on my back, including food supplies.

Once I got to La Compañía, the people fled when I appeared. Even the dogs disappeared with their tails between their legs, as though I were some kind of demon. I greeted every person I saw with "*Allianchu*," the Quechua word for "hello," but it made no difference.

The people treated me with fear and hostility, suspicious of my motives for wanting to live among them. They looked at the ground as I walked by. At times I feared for my life and wondered if I had made a big mistake choosing this community.

From Pilar, the itinerant schoolteacher, I learned that the leader of the community had told the people to forbid their children to speak to me. He had cautioned them that surely I could not have come just to learn Quechua and that I must have some other motive, such as converting them or stealing from them.

A few days after I moved into the dilapidated hacienda, that same leader of the community organized a meeting. All the heads of families voted to kick me out, saying that I was surely "an agent of the devil." Pilar spoke passionately on my behalf. She had much influence and respect among the people. By the end of the meeting, the leader changed his mind and permitted me to stay.

Initially, the only ones who spoke to me were the drunks. A drunken woman came up to me and said something in Quechua in a menacing voice. Not understanding her words but seeing her toothless sneer, I could only imagine the horrible things she was saying to me.

During that first terrifying week, three drunken men approached the courtyard of the hacienda and shouted that they wanted something to eat. I brought out some fresh bread I had baked in the little oven I had made by placing a large tin can over the wood stove. I cut a slice for each of the men. The spokesman for the group told the men not to eat the bread. He turned to me and demanded that I eat it first.

Pilar later explained that they thought I might have bewitched the bread or poisoned it. Of course, I ate my slice, showing what I thought were convincing signs of great relish. The drunken spokesman was not convinced. He asked me in broken Spanish, "What's in it?" I began to list milk, eggs… He broke in with a sinister look on his face, "I don't see any milk or eggs. You're lying. There's just wheat in this bread. Show me the milk and eggs." I was convinced he was going to attack me.

Fortunately, an old Indigenous man happened to be walking home up the mountain. As he passed by, he saw what was going on in the courtyard and barked at the men in Quechua. They immediately became docile, hid their bread under their ponchos, and looked at the ground. I used this opportunity to make a quick exit. I took some deep, slow breaths to relieve the tension in my body.

A similar experience happened during that same week on a Saturday, just as it was becoming night. I was in my room lighting the candles when I heard someone walk into the house. The hacienda had no front door, so I had hung a thick piece of fabric in the doorway—but it obviously wasn't enough to stop an intruder. I went to the front room and saw a man standing in the doorway. Through the window I spotted the dark shapes of four other men. Fear gripped my insides and made my heart pound in my chest.

These young men were not from La Compañía. They had probably come from Cusubamba, a town an hour away by foot. It was hard to tell if they were Indians or poor Mestizos, the distinction being very small where I lived.

I gathered up all my courage and stood in the man's path so he couldn't enter any further. I crossed my arms, mimicking a pose of self-confidence, and forced myself to bark the Spanish equivalent of "Just what the hell do you think you're doing in my house?"

The man in the doorway said, with a threatening smile, "Just looking around." One of the men outside said mockingly, "Doesn't the Señorita want to practice her Quechua with us?"

I felt paralyzed with fear, but managed to function by mimicking a person who is self-assured—a skill I'd learned while climbing in the mountains. I threatened them with everything I could think of, saying that if they didn't leave this minute I would tell the priest, the police, and their bosses to make sure they'd lose their jobs in Quito. The guy in the doorway turned around and walked outside, making sure to take his time. I didn't wait to see where they went.

After the men left, I pushed two heavy pieces of furniture against the open front doorway to impede entry. I passed a sleepless night with my hunting knife at my side, a gift from a Navajo friend.

Those were hard times for me. Fortunately, they only lasted about ten days, thanks to the influence of Pilar, the schoolteacher. Gradually, as the days wore on, the hostility of the people turned to simple shyness. One day, as I walked home from the Wednesday market in Cusubamba, I sucked on a fruit called *sapote*. A young girl about 12 years old passed me, driving her pigs to the market. I offered her a piece of fruit. She seemed very pleased. I told her to come and get it. She said no. She finally told me to put it on the ground. She still didn't come and get it. Clearly she was afraid of me, so I walked away. I looked back and saw her run up and grab the fruit and run a few yards down the mountain. When she was quite far away, she shouted, "*Qué Dios lo pagui*," broken Spanish for "May God repay you."

From that experience, I learned to use fruit to lure the children to come closer and closer to me. They grabbed the fruit and ran away. It was typically the girls who showed the most bravery. After a few days of leaving a piece of fruit on the ground with decreasing distance between the fruit and me, I finally placed an orange in my lap. The bravest of the girls crawled into my lap, took the orange, and bit into it while the juice ran down her smiling face. From that moment, the children lost their shyness.

The adults' shyness continued to wear away as I worked side by side with the people in the *mingas*—community work days in which everyone contributes his or her service to better the area, a custom dating from the time of the Incas. During the first few work days, I joined the men in building Pilar's new schoolhouse. The men tolerated my ignorance in matters related to building and let me feel like I was actually helping them.

Within a mere three weeks, the people had made a complete turnaround in their attitude toward me. Almost every day I got several invitations for lunch in one of the *chozas*, the mud-bricked, thatch-roofed houses that dot the side of the mountain.

Lunch was usually a thick soup called *mazamorra*, slowly cooked in a huge caldron suspended over the fire. The soup contained every kind of edible plant that was cultivated in the area, including barley, quinoa, potatoes, onions, and sometimes corn. The soup often served as both breakfast and lunch. The people didn't eat much meat. They sold their sheep and pigs at a nearby market to make extra money. They also raised guinea pigs inside their homes and ate them only on special occasions, like a marriage or other celebration.

Men and women began coming to my house to talk of their troubles. They told me how angry they were because they discovered that the landowner—my landlord—paid them much lower than the minimum wage mandated by law of 50 cents a day. I could have easily told them that they had the right to make a legal complaint in Quito at the office of land reform, but I was too afraid my landlord would find out I was causing trouble. I simply lent a sympathetic ear to the people.

The next time the landowner came to pay the people's monthly wages, a group representing the entire community came to him and told him they were angry and were not going to work anymore if he didn't raise their wages. The very next day he doubled their wages to 40 cents a day. Maybe the landowner feared being killed, similar to what had happened to a landowner from the same general area a decade before. Thankfully, he didn't accuse me of causing the commotion.

Over time, I began to regard the little room I had in the hacienda as rather nice, just a bit on the dark side. I had a bed, chest of drawers, cupboard, and table, plus the wood stove with my improvised metal oven on top. That room served as my refuge when times were rough with the people during the first few weeks.

The rat situation was depressing, however. These particular rats were a large variety—about the size of a small cat. They were bold and even came out during the day. Sometimes I stayed awake at night for fear they would jump onto my bed. I put out poison. After a few days, none of the rats ate it anymore. They are smart animals and learn quickly.

One night, after an especially frustrating day, while I was reading in my bed with the candles lit, a huge rat waddled across the straw mat toward my bed. I made a noise, hoping to frighten it away. It kept coming. Something broke inside of me and out came a flood of tears, accompanied by all the strongest insults I could think of in Spanish, Quechua, and English, along with a book I threw at the rat. My fury took me by surprise.

I slept well that night, relieved of my pent-up frustration and anxiety. Like everything else, the rat situation improved radically over time. I followed the suggestion of another Peace Corps volunteer and put steel wool in all the holes. At night I tightly secured the thick fabric that served as my front door by placing a chest of drawers firmly against the two door jambs.

The water, on the other hand, continued to be a problem. I had to haul every drop of water from the irrigation ditch about 100 yards above the hacienda. The water appeared dark and muddy. After filtering and boiling, it took on a yellow hue and tasted like dirt.

The house had no toilet, or so I thought. I relieved myself in a hidden nook in the fields, like everyone else around there. With an old metal bowl I found on one of the shelves, I dug a makeshift latrine and then left the bowl nearby to throw dirt into the little pit after each use. Scraggly, malnourished dogs gathered every morning outside, waiting for me to relieve myself. As soon as I walked away from the latrine, the dogs eagerly dug up the fecal feast. "Why mine?" I wondered. I speculated that it had something to do with the relatively high nutritional content—or maybe they simply preferred the foreign flavor.

After a few weeks of living in this community, I discovered that I had dead roundworms a foot long in my stools. The thought of harboring worms thoroughly disgusted me, yet the latent scientist in me also found the worms fascinating. I wanted to show my Peace Corps friends these creatures. I got a stick and pulled out the two longest worms I could find, rinsed them off, and laid the fat, pink-colored worms out on the porch railing. I forgot about the sun, which made them shrivel into the size of earthworms, not worthy of show-and-tell.

The Peace Corps office gave me de-worming pills, similar to the kind veterinarians give to dogs. The nurse informed me that the scientific term for this type of roundworm was *Ascaris lumbicoides*. She said that many of the Peace Corps volunteers in Ecuador had sought treatment for Ascaris worms. I had to take two courses of the worm medication during my stay on the mountain. Without running water, maintaining proper hygiene posed quite a challenge.

During his monthly visit, the *hacendado,* incredulous that I had remained in La Compañía, unlocked a room adjacent to my bedroom. I had assumed the locked room was used for storing items. Instead, the room, the size of a closet, contained a toilet. At last, a real toilet! Every day, I hauled a bucket of water from the irrigation ditch to flush the toilet.

My project in La Compañía primarily focused on recording children telling local legends in Quechua, which would later be made into a Quechua-Spanish textbook to be used in bilingual schools. Pilar agreed to help me transcribe the recordings and translate them into Spanish. She also agreed to help me put together a dictionary of the local dialect with Spanish translation.

Once the children no longer feared me—and my tape recorder—they loved to come and tell me stories in Quechua about their lives. The girls would sit in my lap. The boys showed more reserve and stood nearby. I recorded them as they spoke, then played the recording back to them. They squealed with wonder and delight and looked at each other with disbelief. Of course I didn't understand much of the stories they recounted, but I felt the children's excitement when they heard themselves speaking. They took turns holding the tape recorder. They turned it over in their hands as though looking for the source of the magic.

Every time Pilar returned to the community, she listened to the tape recordings and then transcribed the stories onto paper. The final step involved translating the stories into Spanish. After a few months, we had accumulated almost enough stories for a book. We intended to have Quechua on one side of the page and Spanish on the other when our little textbook would be published someday in Quito—we hoped.

For my project, the Peace Corps provided me with not only a portable tape recorder to record legends, but also a Polaroid camera. The first photo I took caused quite a commotion of excitement. The children watched, dumbstruck, as the images began to appear. One of the boys, Julio, took the photo and turned it around and around, trying to make sense out of what he saw emerging, as the rest of the children looked over his shoulder. A girl squealed and pointed to the image of Julio in the photo. Since the villagers didn't have mirrors to look at themselves, Julio did not believe that the image was of him. Then all the children got involved in figuring out who the rest of the people were in the photo.

One day a few weeks into my stay, a young boy invited me to eat lunch in his *choza*. Juan had befriended me and became one of my informants for the future bilingual textbook. He told me that he lived with his mother and his baby sister, Marta, who had gotten sick. He said she would probably die. His mother didn't have any money to take the baby to a doctor.

Juan told me his father had died a few months ago after he got drunk and fell off a wall doing construction work in Quito. After he died, Juan's brother left home at the age of 12 to look for work in Quito to support the family.

It broke my heart hearing these stories. Life was so hard for these people. I wondered how they could endure such hardships. Juan was ten years old and in the first grade at the community school. He had to delay entering school because his mother needed his help at home. Juan told me his mother cried every night because she was so scared that something would happen to the older boy who supported the family. She feared their family would starve to death.

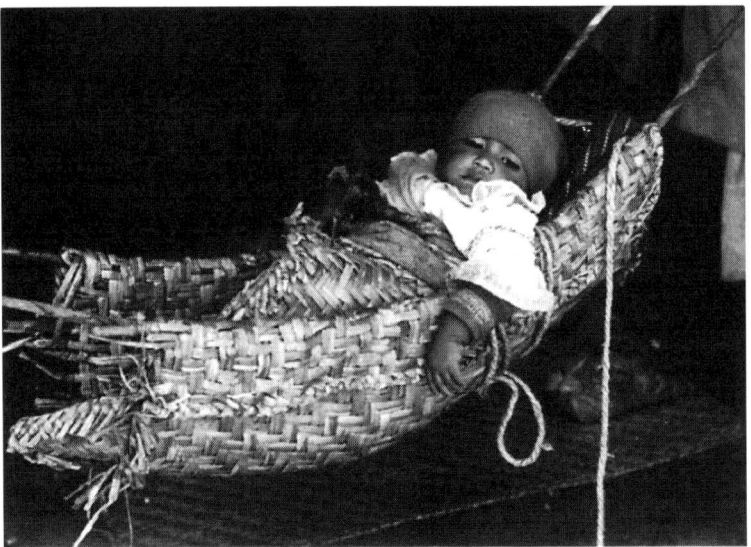

Sick baby in a woven hammock

I brought the family some of my food. I also brought an aspirin from my first aid kit. I crushed the aspirin and then gave the mother a tiny grain to give to her sick baby. I said the benediction while making the sign of the cross on the baby's forehead. The next day the mother told me via her son that the baby was healed. I didn't believe that an aspirin could heal a sick baby. I thought it must be a coincidence.

After that, mothers brought me their sick babies so I could "heal" them. I felt like a fake, but somehow the babies seemed to get well pretty quickly. I spent a lot of time wondering about the seemingly miraculous healings. I recognized that there was some kind of healing force at work, but it was not coming from me or from my crushed grains of aspirin or my phony benedictions. But, on second thought, maybe my fervent intention to help the babies and their mothers made some sort of difference. In that era, I had never heard of the word "placebo."

The mothers brought me roasted guinea pigs on sticks as thank-you presents. The idea of eating these little animals that looked like skewered rats brought on waves of nausea, but I ate them anyway, remembering the admonitions of the Peace Corps officials to accept food when it was offered.

The day after I visited Juan and his mother, the young boy called Julio came to my hacienda and called out to me, saying that his mother wanted me to come for lunch. We walked far down the mountain and over a hill to reach his *choza* compound. All the *chozas* looked the same to my untrained eye. They each had just one large square room, with adobe walls, a roof of straw tied to a frame, and a dirt floor. There were no windows, only a hole for the smoke to escape. Two *chozas* in each compound stood beside each other at right angles. One was used for cooking and storing and as a general work area. The other was for sleeping. Each family had their own compound.

Julio held my hand as he guided me inside the *choza*. I could see nothing until my eyes adjusted to the dim light. I smelled the soup simmering in an immense, blackened pot that hung from a metal stand over a fire in the center of the room. Julio's younger sister stirred the pot continuously as the food cooked, while his younger brother played outside.

All the walls were lined with an assortment of earthen jugs with grains and corn inside. A straw mat hammock supported by branches served as a bed for somebody—or several people. A pair of chaps made of sheepskin hung from a pole.

We ate our soup cross-legged on the floor. I used every opportunity to insert a word or phrase I knew in Quechua. I said, *Simaq mikhuna*. Delicious food. After a pause, I added, *sulpayki*. Thank you.

After we ate, and after I had asked the names of all the objects I saw in the *choza*, we went outside and sat among the stalks of harvested barley to enjoy the sunny day. While I admired the view of the valley below, the three children gathered around to explore my body. They began with my head: Carmencita thoroughly searched my hair for lice. She made many little parts to expose my scalp.

The children asked me endless questions, like where was my husband and where were my children, and why was my skin white and theirs dark. The priest was the only other white person who had ever lived in their community. In answer to the skin-color question, I pointed to one of their black guinea pigs and then pointed to a tan-colored guinea pig. The children smiled and gave understanding nods. When they got tired of asking questions, they continued examining my body.

Carmencita brought out all her ribbons, her comb carved from horn, and a pail of water. She made dozens of little braids in my hair. After her hair styling was finished, she stood back to assess her work. She didn't like what she saw and undid the braids. Then all three kids ran their hands over my arms, commenting on each mole or freckle, scar, and vein.

When their explorations brought them to my chest, they talked about my breasts without a trace of embarrassment. Among the Indigenous people of that area, breasts did not seem to be sexual symbols as they are in American culture. It was common to see women walking about with their breasts partly or all the way exposed, even when they were not nursing.

Julio cupped his hands and reached for my breasts very innocently. Then he asked if he could see them. The request took me by surprise. I said I'd rather not open my blouse. Carmencita paid no attention to what I said to Julio. She opened the top two buttons and peeped down my blouse and then reached her hand in and squeezed. "No milk," she announced. She asked if she could suck on them anyway. It took me a few moments to mentally process that strange interaction.

I had occasionally seen children as old as ten suck on their mother's breasts, but now my own breasts were the object of attention! I said "No" to Carmencita's request, explaining that I didn't want to open my blouse. She said I didn't need to open my blouse. She started to suck with the blouse and all, making loud sucking sounds. The shock of her action left me speechless. Eventually I regained my wits and asked her to stop.

Her sucking left a big wet area on my blouse that made me look like a breast-feeding mother who had leaked milk from her nipples. I felt very strange.

When the children got tired of looking me over, we went to the edge of the *choza* to watch Carmencita make a *shigra*, a woven bag made out of plant fibers. As she was teaching me, we conversed in elementary Quechua, since practicing, after all, was the main object of my visit. The children intermittently sprinkled Spanish words throughout their conversations. I understood only the gist of what the children said to me.

As the afternoon wore on, it became time for me to walk back up the mountain and work on transcribing the legends I had gathered. As I left, I said, *rutukama, guambra*. Goodbye, children.

On Wednesdays I walked to market, an hour away in Cusubamba. On the path I met many Indians heading in the same direction. Market day was a happy day for most, because it gave the people a chance to get away, see friends, gossip, look at merchandise in the little plaza, relax, and get drunk.

The first time I walked to the market, I watched a truck slowly lumber down the road, heading in my direction. A familiar face looked down and yelled for me to jump aboard. I ran behind the slow-moving truck, threw my empty pack on board, grabbed a metal handrail, and struggled to hoist myself up. Several people leaned over and grabbed various parts of my body, pulling me up and into the truck. The people smiled and laughed, finding me to be quite entertaining.

We all stood cramped tightly together along with four pigs and a cow that the *campesinos* intended to sell in the plaza. After getting to the market and chatting among the buyers and sellers, I lugged my heavy pack back home, laden with food for the week.

The Peace Corps office asked me to write a series of articles about my time in La Compañía for their monthly newsletters. In an excerpt from one of the many articles, I wrote, "From where I live, I can see the whole valley stretch away below me. In the evening, if I wait patiently, I can see the snow-covered volcanoes as the clouds drift past, including Cotopaxi, Iliniza, and Quilindaña. At night I see the tiny lights of Salcedo in the far distance. It is a peaceful area. The Indians are friendly to me. I am happy here."

After a couple months of spending almost all my time in La Compañía, I began to miss my climbing friends and our adventures in the high mountains. The following weekend, I hiked down the mountain to the paved road, caught the bus to Quito, and picked up my two checks at the Peace Corps office, $120 per month. From the office, I telephoned Mateo, my mountaineering friend, and the best friend of Jorge. We made a plan to meet up. I couldn't wait to see him after the long absence.

Chapter 21

MY FRIEND MATEO

MATEO MET ME IN DOWNTOWN QUITO on a Saturday and asked if I would like to meet his family. He let me know that they were poor and lived in a humble part of town.

Because Mateo had exceptional intelligence, the government had given him a full merit scholarship to attend the National Polytechnic University in Quito. Mateo's family pinned their hopes on him, with the expectation that he would eventually take them out of desperate poverty.

When I asked Mateo how he first got involved in the school's climbing club, he said that the club provided plenty of good food for the climbers on the weekends when they climbed. He knew he would have a respite from gnawing hunger during those outings. He didn't anticipate that he would soon get hooked on mountaineering and become one of Ecuador's most accomplished climbers.

After listening to Mateo's story, I suggested we visit the outdoor market and buy food to contribute to the midday meal at his home. While we were buying vegetables and other ingredients for the meal, I looked at all the live animals in cages. I saw a young turkey in a little cage made of sticks. I thought the turkey would make a sweet little pet for the family and bought it.

Mateo's mother and sister were polite to me but shy and reserved.

They seemed pleased with the gifts, especially the young turkey, which they let out of the cage. The turkey walked around exploring the house. After a few minutes it disappeared.

After about an hour had passed, Mateo's mother called us to the table. She served a delicious stew. The meat had a familiar taste that I recognized. I asked where the little turkey was. Everyone at the table laughed out loud at my naïveté. After a few seconds, I laughed along with them and acknowledged my ignorance. I thanked them for sharing the delicious soup with me.

That afternoon we wandered around the city and hung out in the park. We talked about life and about Jorge. I shared the little information I knew from the letters Jorge wrote to me about his day-to-day life in Hungary.

When I told Mateo that I planned to remain loyal to Jorge during the three or four years he was in Hungary, he asked me a simple question: "Do you plan to stay in Ecuador until Jorge returns?" At that moment, I fully comprehended the unlikelihood that I would remain in Ecuador after my service in the Peace Corps ended. I quickly pushed that thought out of my mind and answered, "I don't know."

Mateo asked if I wanted to spend the next day together visiting the picturesque town of Otavalo. We could climb an extinct volcano called Imbaburo, an easy day climb not far from the town.

That night, I returned to the private home where I stayed while in Quito. The next morning, Mateo and I met at the bus station and traveled north for two hours to reach our destination. Before exploring the town, we climbed Imbaburo. Mateo said that the Otavalo people had a spiritual relationship with the mountain. They referred to it as *Taita Imbabura*, or "Papa Imbabura," and viewed it as the sacred protector of the region. At a little over 15,000 feet above sea level, the volcano had no glaciers, only snowfields near the summit, making technical equipment unnecessary.

Grazing cows and crops of sugarcane and beans covered the lower slopes of Imbabura. The farmers also grew maize, a type of corn that the people used as feed for animals. Volcanic ash from former eruptions covered the mountainside, contributing to the richness of the soil and the lushness of the crops.

The relative wealth and elegant clothing of the Otavalo people contrasted sharply with the extreme poverty of Indigenous communities elsewhere. The men wore spotless white calf-length pants and dark, hand-woven ponchos. A long, single braid hung down their backs, with a fedora hat perched on their heads. The women and girls wore dark woolen skirts and white blouses with colorful embroidery and woven waistbands. Both men and women wore their hair in braids.

Much of the wealth of the Otavalo people came from selling their distinctive weavings and folk art in the markets throughout the town. Mateo told me that some of the Otavalo men travel around the world selling their famous handicrafts.

While we meandered through the many folk art markets near the center of town, I listened to the hauntingly beautiful Andean panpipe folk music in the background, played by several groups of musicians.

At the end of the day, we took the bus back to Quito. A current of sadness ran through me when it was time to leave Mateo and return to La Compañía de Jesús Cristo. We agreed to meet the next few weekends to climb together. Back home in La Compañía, when I wasn't occupied with visiting families, gathering folk legends, and doing my daily chores, I found myself daydreaming about climbing with Mateo in the mountains.

The following weekend I came a day early to Quito to do some errands. Consuelo, the owner of the house where I stayed, had given me the key to the front door and told me I could come and go as I pleased whenever I came into town. When I stayed at her home, I took advantage of the opportunity to take long showers. What a thrill to feel the water pour over me and to get completely clean! But, on that particular day, something strange happened while I took my shower.

After luxuriating under the showerhead for a longer stretch of time than usual, I began to feel lightheaded for no apparent reason. I remember getting out of the shower and reaching for the towel. After that, I don't remember anything except waking up on a bed. Consuelo and her son were leaning over me, looking distraught and frantic. A thin blanket lay over my naked body.

I heard a siren outside the house. A man in a blue uniform came into the house and gave me oxygen to breathe with a mask. He lifted my barely conscious body and gently placed it on a gurney that he wheeled outside. He slid the gurney and me into the back of an ambulance parked beside the house. With the help of the supplemental oxygen, my brain began to function again. As we drove to the hospital with the siren blaring, I became fully aware of my surroundings and what people were saying to me, as though I was waking from a very deep sleep.

The neurologist on duty at the main hospital in Quito escorted me from the ambulance into the ER. He shined a light into my eyes to make sure the pupils constricted normally, checked my reflexes, and then asked me questions to test my mental status. Although I felt confused and nauseated, and I had a bad headache, I managed to answer the questions correctly—but only after long pauses. The neurologist pronounced me "stable" and requested that I stay overnight for observation. I asked him what happened. He said I had carbon monoxide poisoning from the poorly ventilated gas water heater in the bathroom of the house where I stayed. As he spoke, I remembered that the tiny bathroom had no windows.

Consuelo drove to the hospital and filled me in on the details of what happened. She said that when she came home from work in the afternoon, she saw her 11-year-old son standing in the bathroom doorway, paralyzed with fright. She looked into the bathroom and saw my naked body on the floor. I was unconscious.

Consuelo knew immediately that I'd been poisoned by carbon monoxide. The gas water heater in the bathroom had a problem with incomplete combustion. She'd intended to get it fixed but hadn't gotten around to it. She'd forgotten to tell me not to use the shower.

She and her traumatized son dragged me out of the bathroom and hoisted me onto the bed in the next room. When Consuelo recounted what happened, I couldn't help imagining the shock that her son experienced from seeing a naked woman's body—not to mention a half-dead naked woman.

After spending the night in the hospital, I called Mateo to let him know I wouldn't be climbing with him that weekend. I wanted to recuperate at home in La Compañía. I would see him the following weekend. Mateo expressed his concern over my near loss of life, but I reassured him that I had made a good recovery.

I didn't know much about carbon monoxide poisoning. The neurologist explained that the carbon monoxide gas replaced some of the oxygen in my red blood cells, essentially starving my body of adequate oxygen. He said it might take several weeks until my body would produce enough new red blood cells to raise my energy and clear my mind.

I didn't want to wait several weeks to feel better. Intuitively, I did a lot of heavy exercise, reasoning that the remaining oxygen would thereby be forced into my cells. I learned years later in my medical training that daily intense exercise improves oxygen uptake from the blood into the cells. Every morning I jogged several miles along the road that ran through the foothills around La Compañía, determined to get over the shortness of breath I was experiencing and get back into shape for climbing.

The people along the road stared at me as I ran past. One man called out in Spanish, "*Señorita*, why are you doing penance?" The people thought surely I must be punishing myself in order to repent for some sin I had committed. I could not convince them that I ran for pleasure, as well as to make myself strong.

During one of my jogs, I saw an old woman herding her sheep barefooted in an area with a light coat of snow on the ground. I wondered how she could withstand the cold. I stopped, took off my shoes and socks, and tried jogging in the snow. At first my feet stung from the cold; then they became like blocks of wood. I finally gave up and put my socks and shoes back on, wondering how I could make my feet tough enough to withstand the cold like the old woman.

One day, after I returned from a strenuous weekend of climbing, a boy I had befriended saw that I was limping. He asked me what was wrong with my foot. I took off my running shoe and showed him the big toe on my right foot. It was red and swollen, with some pus oozing from the inner edge of the nail bed. The front of my climbing boot had pressed on the toenail and caused it to become ingrown. I had soaked my foot in hot, salty water, with little improvement. The boy told me to follow him to the "doctor."

The village "doctor" looked like a wild man. His hair was disheveled and he smelled of alcohol. As he examined my toe, he said something in Quechua, which the boy translated into Spanish. "The doctor says you must sit down and give him your foot. He will make the problem go away. But first you must drink a cup of *chicha*."

Chicha is a fermented beer made from corn that is chewed up by the women and spit into a large pot with a few spices. The saliva contains enzymes that help turn the corn into sugar, which then ferments into alcohol. I was familiar with this custom from having lived with traditional Navajo people who chewed corn for making special bread for their puberty ceremonies. Nevertheless, this chewed corn felt different. I forced myself to drink a few gulps of the *chicha*, enough to feel a slight buzz.

The "doctor" pointed off in the distance and told me to look at a long-tailed red bird flying in the sky. Just as I turned my head, I felt a searing pain that caused me to give a loud yelp, followed by curse words in Spanish and English. I looked at my toe in shock.

The "doctor" had removed my entire toenail with a pair of pliers. While I stared in horror at my toe, the "doctor" poured a little cane alcohol onto the raw and bloody nail bed, provoking another yelp from me. He bound the toe with a strip of fabric and told me to leave it on for two days and then take it off. He told me it would heal quickly and the nail would re-grow over time, which it did.

The "doctor" held out his upturned hand, a gesture indicating that he expected to be paid. I had mixed feelings about the payment. He had removed my toenail without my permission. On the other hand, I recognized that I was in a different culture with different expectations from what I was used to. I asked the boy how to repay the "doctor." He said the "doctor" would probably like some money to buy more alcohol. Instead of giving money that would be spent on alcohol, I told him I was going to make something especially for him. I went home and made the "doctor" two loaves of bread in my makeshift oven. Receiving them, he gave me a big smile, revealing a shiny, gold-covered front tooth.

By the following week the nail bed had healed. I was back in shape mentally and physically, and ready to climb with Mateo. On my way to meet him, I stopped by the post office in Quito to pick up the package my parents had sent me after I asked for some expensive climbing equipment, including high-quality boots, crampons, and a climbing rope. I spent half a day at the post office, overcoming administrative obstacles and filling out forms, only to discover that the package had been stolen.

When I told Mateo about the loss, he told me not to worry because he knew of a way to get the best possible equipment, and it wouldn't cost us any money. He said that climbing expeditions from Europe and the United States often contacted the climbing club looking for local guides. In lieu of payment, the guides accepted some of the foreigners' state-of-the-art climbing equipment that the climbers wouldn't need after they left Ecuador. He suggested that we go to the club and see if there was a group in need of a guide.

By chance, just as we arrived at the club, a Swiss expedition drove up in a van. Mateo and I offered to be their guides on Cotopaxi, the volcano they wanted to climb to get in shape before attempting more difficult climbs. They eagerly accepted our offer.

I had fun interacting with the four Swiss men. They were playful with me. I let them know I was half Swiss. One of them asked, "Which half?" We spoke in a mixture of German, English—and Spanish so Mateo could understand what we were saying. Occasionally I threw in a Swiss phrase from my childhood, which made the Swiss men smile.

While we hiked to the trailhead, the men wanted to know if I was afraid when I climbed on the glaciers in the high mountains. "Yes, of course I'm afraid," I said. "I'm terrified, but I do it anyway." I told them I was training myself to be mentally and physically strong and brave for what might lie ahead in my life. The Swiss men looked puzzled by my response. It would have taken too long to tell them about the Navajo grandmother's prophecy.

What I didn't mention to the Swiss men is that, when I'm climbing mountains, I discover aspects of myself I didn't know I had. On one of my climbs with Mateo, I discovered the power of my imagination, which helped me survive a potentially life-threatening situation.

One time Mateo and I had gotten completely lost on the broad summit of one of the volcanoes. A raging snowstorm caused a rapid buildup of snow that obliterated our tracks. The total whiteout left us disoriented, without any visible landmarks to guide us. Our headlamps were useless in the whiteout, and neither of us owned a compass.

It was common among my Ecuadorian climbing friends not to own certain equipment that other climbers would consider indispensable. What my friends lacked in equipment they made up for with their mountaineering expertise.

We blindly headed down the mountain, only to discover that we had descended the east side of the mountain into the Amazon jungle. Once we realized our serious mistake, we turned around and headed back up the mountain. Already thoroughly exhausted from ten hours of climbing up the mountain and down the other side, I didn't know how I was going to climb back up the mountain. Each step was an overwhelming effort.

I remember Mateo telling me that he had almost frozen to death during a storm a few years before. Once the fear of dying subsided, he said he felt very peaceful. I imagined myself lying down in the snow and freezing to death—holding on to Mateo's words about freezing being a peaceful experience.

Just as I was on the brink of telling Mateo to go on without me, my mind did something that helped me survive the brutal trek back up the mountain. I conjured in my imagination a vivid scene in which I had to rescue a small child who was crying inconsolably and had nearly frozen to death at the top of the mountain. She had been taken there and left to die. Time was of the essence in saving the child's life.

Being on an imaginary rescue mission gave me energy that seemed to come out of nowhere. Without holding this scenario in my imagination, I could not have kept going in such extreme conditions.

Mateo and I made it back to the top of the mountain—no child anywhere to be seen—and then down the side of our original ascent. At eight o'clock that evening, after 20 hours of climbing, we crawled into our tent and collapsed, grateful to be alive. As I lay in my sleeping bag reflecting on the prior 24 hours, I realized that the force of my mind and imagination is what made it possible for me to climb back up the enormous mountain—instead of giving in to the limitations of my physical body, lying down in the snow, and freezing to death. I never told Mateo how I managed to survive that ordeal.

Throughout my life's journey, I've discovered that being of service to people in need—even if the service is purely imaginary—is what feeds my soul and sustains me in challenging times.

When Mateo and I fulfilled our role as guides on Cotopaxi, the Swiss men expressed their gratitude and exhilaration. They promised that before they returned to Switzerland, and after they finished their climbs in Ecuador, they would give their beautiful Swiss climbing rope to Mateo, plus some warm gloves and a pair of goggles to me as payment. I could have felt like Mateo got a better deal, but I realized that the goggles were exactly what I needed.

In those days, I frequently burned my corneas, even when wearing homemade goggles, due to the intensity of the sunlight reflecting off the high-altitude glaciers. When I moved my eyes, it felt like I had ground glass in them. I would have to lie in bed for a whole day with my eyes shut in Consuelo's apartment, waiting for the corneas to heal. Mateo would come by and check up on me, giving me advice and words of encouragement.

All my climbing companions used homemade goggles and never suffered from snow blindness the way I did. They said that people with blue eyes, and green eyes like mine, were at higher risk of snow blindness than people with brown eyes, who had more protective pigment in the iris. The Swiss goggles helped prevent further damage to my eyes.

Along with my eyes, my skin took a beating too. Before the advent of sunscreen, burns were inevitable. I sustained some serious burns on my face before I learned more about what precautions to take while climbing on the glaciers. The first time I got a bad burn, the top layer of skin came off in thin sheets. I had a fright when I saw myself in the mirror at Consuelo's place. The "doctor" in La Compañía gave me some herbal concoctions to drink and to put on my skin. They made the burns heal quickly without any scars. I never forgot about how powerful herbal medicine can be.

Chapter 22

FROM PARADISE TO REVOLUTION

MATEO AND I TOOK SOME UNFORGETTABLE TRIPS together on the weekends and during holidays. I covered the costs. Although I made only $120 per month, I was wealthy compared to what Mateo had to live on, which was practically nothing.

One three-day weekend, we took a long bus ride to Colombia, the country north of Ecuador. No one had warned us that Colombia, in those days, could be a dangerous place for travelers—especially travelers camping in tents. In our campground on the beach, we heard about two people who'd been robbed at gunpoint while in their tents. We spent the following night in a cheap hotel.

The next day, Mateo and I decided to rent horses and ride into the jungle. After we'd been riding for about an hour, a man on horseback galloped toward us, holding a gun in his hand pointed at us. He demanded our money. I happened to have a couple of US dollar bills in my little change purse that I gave him. He seemed pleased and rode off. We didn't have much for people to steal. We had very few possessions other than our tent, backpacks, and sleeping bags, which we had left in our hotel. Mateo remained unusually calm after the incident, maybe because he had a lot of experience facing danger. Unlike him, I felt extremely agitated and wanted to get out of the jungle as fast as our horses could gallop.

The next day Mateo and I took a bus to a remote area to visit some ruins. We immersed ourselves in exploring the landscape. When we returned to the parking area, we discovered that the last bus back to the city had already left. We saw only one car parked in the area. The two men in the car saw us and offered us a ride back to the city. Mateo accepted eagerly. I had some fleeting doubts about accepting the ride, but we had no alternative.

Mateo and I sat in the back seat. We rode in silence for the first few miles. I felt a sense of foreboding. I sorely regretted our decision to accept the ride, even though it looked like we didn't have a choice.

The man in the front on the passenger side turned around and smiled at me, exposing a gold-covered tooth. His smile looked sinister and gave me a sense of imminent danger.

The driver lit a cigarette. The smell of smoke filled the car. I rolled down the window to get some fresh air. At that moment I started to feel trapped. It was getting dark outside. I saw only an occasional car on the road.

After about a half-hour of tension-filled silence, both men began asking Mateo questions about me. They recognized that I was a *gringa* and assumed that I didn't speak Spanish. At first the questions were benign, like what country did I come from, and was I Mateo's girlfriend. Then the questions began to get malignant.

I heard the gold-toothed man offer Mateo a large sum of money to "buy" me. At that point, a powerful force inside of me took over. I burst into the conversation with a torrent of curse words in Spanish and said that Mateo and I were about to get married in Bogotá the next day. I lied that Mateo's father was a policeman and my father worked for the CIA.

The men shut up and drove in silence. I thought maybe they planned to kill Mateo and then rape me. I barely breathed for the rest of the ride. I whispered, "Should we jump out of the car?" Mateo thought it was a bad idea. He held my hand tightly. I noticed a tension in his face that I had never seen before.

Fortunately, the men dropped us off at the nearest bus station. I was so rattled, I told Mateo, "I want to go home right now." Going home meant returning to Ecuador. He agreed with the plan.

After a few weeks, Mateo and I embarked on a different kind of adventure during my annual two-week holiday. Mateo told me about a military cargo plane that would take us for free to the Galápagos Islands on one of its twice-weekly trips to deliver supplies. Mateo had never flown in an airplane. I could sense the excitement behind his calm, even temperament.

Nothing, not even looking at photos and reading Darwin's notebooks, could have prepared me for what I saw on the Galápagos Islands—a true paradise with exotic flora and fauna, undisturbed by the ravages of civilization.

I learned from the park ranger that about 10 million years ago, the Pacific Ocean floor exploded with a burst of volcanic activity, resulting in dozens of barren volcanic islands. The Spanish explorers in the 1500s reported seeing countless giant tortoises on the islands. They named the islands *Galápagos*, a Spanish word for a certain species of tortoise.

The landscape appeared otherworldly, with its lava flows, craters, volcanoes, and cacti. And because the islands were so isolated from the rest of the world, some strange species of animals developed—animals not found elsewhere, like blue-footed boobies and giant tortoises.

All the islands except four were uninhabited by humans and protected as a national park. The creatures lived in extraordinary harmony. The fauna were utterly innocent and without fear. They approached us with curiosity—including the birds. One alighted on my arm and then drank out of my water cup. Iguanas ate the cactus flowers we fed them with our hands. We got a glimpse of what the world must have been like before domination and extermination by man in the name of civilization.

We rented a fishing boat and split the cost among four other people hailing from France, England, and Ecuador. We sailed from island to island, exploring and marveling at the wonders. We swam and played with seals and sea lions. We watched as a young child rode on top of a giant land turtle.

I fed a dead lizard to a magnificent hawk that stood right next to me on a black volcanic rock. With his head tilted to one side, he stared at me. We made eye contact. I couldn't tell if that moment lasted a few seconds or a few minutes. It felt like a moment of eternity.

Our boat cruised alongside whales, sharks, sea turtles, and dolphins. We lived on rice and the fish we caught. In the cove where we anchored the boat each evening, the clarity of the greenish-blue water allowed us to see all the way to the bottom of the ocean.

One evening while I swam in the cove, a huge fish approached and swam alongside me. At that moment, I heard people on the boat yelling frantically, "Shark!" My heart pounded furiously as I swam to the side of the boat. Three people reached out and grabbed my life jacket and hauled me on board. The fisherman remained calm. He told me that I had swum with a sand shark, mostly harmless to humans.

The sleeping area in the fishing boat was a tiny space below deck. We had to fit two people in each of the narrow beds to accommodate all of us on board. My body lay right up against Mateo's lean and muscular body. The electricity between us was palpable, but I tried my best to ignore it, determined to fulfill my oath of fidelity to Jorge. I imagined Mateo had similar thoughts, given that Jorge was his best friend. We kept our thoughts to ourselves that night.

After one week on board the fishing boat, we debarked onto land. Mateo and I spent the second week camping in our tent. We hiked, climbed among the lava rock formations, and marveled at the creatures we saw.

By our second day on land, Mateo and I were ravenous. We hadn't eaten dinner the night before. Without much money to buy food at the one tiny grocery store, we tried to strategize what to eat. We had grown tired of eating fresh-caught fish and rice for every meal.

While we were exploring one of the islands, we encountered a group of former colonists, mostly of Swiss and German descent. Their homes clustered at one end of the island. One of the men saw us wandering around and engaged us in conversation. After I spoke some German with him, he invited us to join his family for dinner.

The park ranger was also a guest at the table. During our conversation, I recognized that the meat on our plates was goat meat. I told my story about how I had butchered and eaten sheep and goats while living on the Navajo Reservation.

The park ranger said that the wild goats on the island were considered "pests." The colonists had brought the goats onto the islands in the previous century, long before the Ecuadorian government had decided to eliminate all non-native flora and fauna, including goats, along with the rats that had traveled as unwelcome passengers on board the sailing ships.

Seeing Mateo's hunting knife attached to his belt, the park ranger said, "You are welcome to catch any wild goat and eat it. The goats on the islands are huge, the size of small ponies." Mateo looked at me enthusiastically and asked if I still remembered how to butcher goats.

In our tent that night, I pondered the thought of butchering a goat. The idea of killing an animal repulsed me, not having had to butcher an animal for a few years. But by afternoon the next day, as hunger overtook us, the idea of butchering seemed less repulsive. Mateo looked at me and asked if I wanted to eat goat meat. I nodded—with some ambivalence.

We waited in the brush until a medium-sized goat wandered in our direction. Mateo jumped out of hiding and pursued the goat until it got tired. He pinned the animal down and then adroitly slit its throat with his hunting knife. A wave of nausea and lightheadedness passed through me, but I felt I had to go through with the bloody procedure.

Mateo built a fire. After I skinned the goat and removed the innards, Mateo cut off a leg, impaled it with a pointed stick, and then roasted it over the fire. I walked to the tiny beach nearby, washed the blood off my hands in the ocean, and said a quick prayer of gratitude for the goat and its meat.

Like starving Neanderthals, we took turns gnawing away at the delicious meat on the leg. Mateo roasted the other leg as food for the next day. We carried the remainder of the goat to the Swiss family for them to eat. They were surprised that we were able to catch the goat and knew how to butcher.

At the end of the two weeks, we said a sad goodbye to paradise and flew back in the same military cargo plane that had brought us to the islands. A soldier on the cargo plane told us to be careful: There was some fighting going on in Quito.

Our trip to Galápagos sharply contrasted with what greeted us when we arrived at the airport in Quito. The streets were almost empty. An eerie feeling of doom came over me. We asked an airport official what was happening. He said, "Ecuador is in midst of a revolution!"

Mateo needed to get home to his family right away. We gave each other a bear hug. "*Te riego que tengas mucho cuidado.*" Mateo begged me to be very careful. As he boarded the city bus, we agreed to meet up the following weekend to spend time together in the mountains.

I had never seen a revolution before. Irresistible curiosity overtook my better judgment. I caught the bus that took me downtown where the heaviest fighting was going on. I watched from the edge of the plaza among a crowd of onlookers. All the chaos and violence seemed confusing and poorly organized—like children running around playing a deadly game.

I suspected that the revolution had erupted because of the severe state of inflation. Prices of essentials had quadrupled since my arrival in Ecuador. A few weeks before the revolution, I wrote my parents, "I'm always broke at the end of the month, but of course I don't starve. Most of my money goes into food, while I skimp on other things, like clothes. The people who are poor are terribly mad about the present economic situation, including the university students. Sometimes I think a revolution is inevitable. I've heard unsubstantiated rumors that a group of university students are training some of the *campesinos* in guerrilla warfare. One thing is certain: The people feel cheated because the government made big promises to them when oil was discovered in the jungle." The premonition I expressed in my letter to my parents had materialized.

I walked along the sidewalk on the edge of the plaza in the midst of a crowd of onlookers. A young soldier, probably a teenager, ran past us in the street. A few seconds later, I heard a loud popping sound, like fireworks. At that same moment, the young soldier dropped to his knees and then fell over onto the road. From a few yards away,

I watched the blood ooze out of the bullet hole in his skull. The horror made me disassociate from my feelings.

As I stood staring dumbfounded at the dead man, a university student standing nearby, with his book bag strapped across his chest, walked over to the dead man and reached down to steal his machine gun. Just as he was making off with the weapon, he received multiple bullets to his head. I could see the contents of his brain—a gruesome, nauseating sight. The high levels of adrenaline in my body kept me from fainting.

Tanks and mounted anti-aircraft guns rolled around the main plaza. A person in the crowd yelled, "Run for cover in the cathedral." And that's what we did. We poured into the cathedral and watched from inside.

The scenes I witnessed became a source of recurring nightmares that lasted for several days, causing me to awaken in the middle of the night in a state of alarm, sometimes even yelling for help.

Ecuador was a dictatorship ruled by a military junta of five generals. Mateo had explained to me that a certain branch of the armed forces wanted to take control. One evil battled against another. Perhaps for that reason, the people didn't seem to care who won the battle. They would be in the same position no matter which general won. I couldn't detect any political idealism.

Some of the onlookers looted and destroyed personal property without any political motives—just getting into the action. I took three photos but didn't dare take more. The crowd was so irrational and volatile that I feared they could turn on me for being a *gringa*. My paranoia came from knowing that the American government had a long history of supporting dictatorships in Central and South America to protect vested interests.

As soon as the shooting subsided, I quickly left the area and walked to Consuelo's house. I called Mateo on the phone. He listened to me relate in great detail what I saw while watching the attempted *coup d'état*. He seemed to have a fatalistic attitude toward the uprising, accepting of whatever happened as though it was preordained. Many of the Indigenous people I worked with had a similar view on all aspects of life. Before we hung up, we confirmed our plans for meeting up.

The rebels were subdued after 24 hours of fighting. The president moved back to the palace, which had been destroyed and vandalized. A friend told me that the president had cried—not for all the lives that were destroyed, but because his cherished personal library had been destroyed. This friend also told me the military gave the young soldiers amphetamines to amp them up for the fight.

The following weekend, Mateo and I caught a ride to the base of Cayambe, a massive volcano covered with snowfields and glaciers, located around 40 miles northeast of Quito. We pitched our tent at the edge of the glacier and lay side by side in our sleeping bags, waiting for our midnight departure, when the snow would be firm and easy to walk on with our crampons.

We talked about aliens and UFOs. Mateo told me that during a few climbs, he'd seen strange, oval-shaped space crafts with rotating lights flying low in the sky. He related this information in a matter-of-fact way, as though it was a well-accepted phenomenon.

After witnessing certain occurrences that defy all reason during Navajo healing ceremonies, I had learned to keep an open mind to all possibilities.

As we lay there, Mateo recounted mountaineering stories, including the time he saw three climbers killed in an avalanche. He tried to rescue them, but they were already dead. "It hurt my heart that I couldn't save these young men," he said. "I think about how much their families suffer. I think about my own family when I climb. My mother and my sister depend on me."

As we talked into the night, I could feel the air becoming thick with sexual tension. I had noted a growing attraction to Mateo for a few months but had managed to suppress my feelings. I could feel his attraction to me as well.

We both tried to ignore our volcanic subterranean rumblings and act like nothing was happening as we lay in our respective sleeping bags. After all, Mateo had a strong allegiance to his best friend. The two of them had accomplished many risky first ascents of peaks in Ecuador, further deepening their bond of friendship. And I had sworn an oath to be faithful to Jorge during his years earning his engineering degree in Hungary. I tried to remember whether Jorge had sworn the same oath of fidelity to me.

I finally could not resist asking Mateo if he had ever "been with a woman." He said that three years prior, when he was 18, he had one miserable experience with a woman—a sex worker. The woman was more interested in reading her comic book than in the paid sexual act. After that encounter, Mateo said he lost interest in pursuing sex with women and preferred devoting himself to his studies and to climbing.

A long silence ensued in the tent. And then the inevitable happened.

I asked Mateo if he would like to have a different kind of sexual experience from the unpleasant one he had endured. He gave a smile that lit up his face. He let go of his naturally shy and deferential nature and expressed eagerness to learn the art of making love from an "older woman with experience." The lovemaking marked the beginning of a new dimension of our friendship. We became even more deeply bonded with each other.

Although I'd broken my oath of fidelity to Jorge, I decided to worry about my guilty conscience later.

Being in love galvanized me with abundant energy, propelling me up the mountain without a huge amount of effort. The exhilaration I felt compelled me to periodically burst into breathless song as I climbed up the glaciers to the top of Cayambe. For the next few days, I smiled incessantly.

When I returned to Consuelo's apartment in Quito, overcome with feelings of guilt, I wrote a carefully thought-out letter to Jorge. I wrote that I had been spending all my free time in the mountains with Mateo—his best friend. I confessed that Mateo and I had developed a deep bond and that I had broken the oath I had made to him before he left for Hungary. I told him how terribly sorry I was to cause him pain and suffering, and that I hoped some day he could forgive me and that we could be friends after the wounds healed.

I confessed to Mateo that I had written to Jorge about our sexual relationship. He understood how important it was for me to tell the truth to Jorge, but he was sad that his betrayal might damage the tight bond the two men had with each other.

Mateo and I continued to climb big mountains on the weekends. On one of our excursions, while lying in the tent, we reminisced about our many memorable climbs together.

Mateo asked me when the exact date of my service in the Peace Corps would end. Hearing that it would be in only a few months, he suggested that we plan to make an expedition to Argentina to climb

Aconcagua, the highest mountain in the Western Hemisphere at just under 23,000 feet. He wanted to spend our last days together on the "roof of the Americas." He thought it would be a fitting way for me to end my time in South America. I had no idea where we would get the funds. Mateo said that he would find a way.

While in Quito a few weeks later, I stopped by the Peace Corps office to pick up my mail. I received a packet from Jorge, my former boyfriend and self-appointed mountaineering coach. Reaching into the packet, I pulled out photos of the two of us, along with dozens of tender love letters that I had written to Jorge over the past year. Jorge wrote that he never wanted to see me ever again and to never write him again and to regard him as dead.

Judging from his intense anger, it was obvious how much pain Jorge suffered from the shattering news about my sexual relationship with Mateo. Remorse washed over me. I wished I had never made that oath to be faithful to Jorge throughout all the years he remained abroad. That was the last time I made that kind of unrealistic promise to anyone.

Chapter 23

AN UNPLANNED EVENT

MY FINAL MONTHS IN ECUADOR took an abrupt turn when my old friend Arthur wrote that he intended to visit me in La Compañía and stay for three weeks. A sickening wave came over me as I remembered something I had tried to forget—a terrifying experience that countless women have endured throughout the world.

Arthur had attended a college in New Hampshire where my father served as dean of students after retiring from the army in 1966. The students viewed my father as a warm and caring father figure. Young men and women often came to the house to volunteer their help with chores in the vegetable and flower gardens or to simply hang out and talk to my parents. Sometimes they would stay for dinner.

During my visits home, I often encountered Arthur spending time with my parents. His bond with them continued long after he had graduated and settled down in a nearby town.

While in New Hampshire visiting, I sometimes spent time alone with Arthur, hiking in the woods or sitting around the wood stove in his cabin, having deep intellectual conversations about life.

Our friendship was purely platonic until one night in my bedroom on the third floor of my parents' home in New Hampshire during the winter holidays in December of 1973. I had returned from the

Navajo Reservation three months before and was preparing for my trip to South America to serve in the Peace Corps.

Arthur came over to say goodbye the evening before my departure. The prolonged goodbye became physical and included a request by Arthur to spend the night with me.

To my horror, I felt my diaphragm dislodge at a critical moment during the act of making love. I had a sinking feeling that I tried to ignore.

On January 2, 1974, I traveled to New Orleans for the Peace Corps Volunteer orientation program. It was too early for me to know if I was pregnant, but just the same, I walked around with a nameless sense of dread.

During our staging, there was a question-and-answer period about anything we might want to know concerning the Peace Corps. To appease my foreboding thoughts, I asked a man from the headquarters in Washington, DC, how the Peace Corps would handle a single woman who became pregnant, trying to sound as casual and theoretical as possible. His succinct answer, "Termination," obviously meant that the volunteer would be sent back home—and not termination of the pregnancy.

What do I do now? A sense of doom swept over me.

After our orientation, our group flew to Quito, where we began classes in language and culture. As the days went by, my excitement over discovering a new country and improving my skills in speaking Spanish became mixed with fear as I waited in vain for my overdue period to come and relieve all the terrible anxiety.

Finally, I took my urine to a lab so that the results would confirm what I already knew from my rapidly swelling breasts and the morning nausea.

When I returned to get the results, the nurse smiled and said, "*Felicitaciones!*"

While my heart pounded furiously in my chest, I took the results and walked out of the building. Only then did I dare look at the piece of paper. The test was positive. All the blood left my head as I staggered toward a bench, where I collapsed into a seated position.

Every morning during this time, I participated robotically in the classes on Spanish language and Ecuadorian culture. I felt isolated from the other volunteers, weighed down by my big secret. I asked myself why I didn't go to the administration, tell them my problem, and insist that they change such an antiquated policy. I knew the answer, though. I feared being terminated from the Peace Corps. Despite my troubles, I had begun enjoying my time in South America.

Abortion is illegal in Ecuador. Finding a doctor who would do the procedure required persistence and a certain amount of artifice. I asked many Ecuadorians for information, trying to act like the question pertained to someone other than me, although surely some of the people I spoke with must have guessed what was really going on. I got many different responses. Some said that they didn't want to give out information and be responsible in case something went wrong. Others talked of the criminal injustice of killing a fetus and the moral obligation of living with one's mistakes. It was not the church-inspired arguments that made me feel like a criminal, but rather, all the sneaking around.

Time was passing. After an emotionally exhausting and frantic search, I enlisted the help of Cindy, a sympathetic Peace Corps volunteer whom I swore to eternal secrecy. With her help, I found a doctor. The name had a familiar sound. Then I remembered the information sheets we'd been given on Ecuador's political parties. The abortionist had been a past presidential candidate of the Communist party.

I made the arrangements by phone. It was early on a dreary Saturday morning when I traveled to Calle Venezuela in downtown Quito. I had told my Ecuadorian family that I was going on a trip for the weekend and wouldn't be back until the following Monday.

After finding the building, I walked through an unlit hallway and up a few flights of stairs. Several women sat in the waiting room, all there for the same purpose, I assumed. After a half-hour wait, a nurse approached me and asked for one thousand *sucres*, the equivalent of $40, one-third of my monthly salary in the Peace Corps. After I handed over the money, she led me to the "operating room."

The doctor came into the small room and told me to undress. I asked him to give me a sheet or something to wrap around my body. He said I didn't need that. Then he told me to use the toilet before the operation. The free-standing toilet stood in a corner of the room with no screen around it to conceal the user. Worse, there was no toilet paper, just a few sheets of newspaper.

The toilet incident marked the beginning of a series of humiliations. I wondered if this man enjoyed being cruel. Was he trying to relieve all his anger toward Americans on me? Was he a misogynist—or simply a mean-spirited person? These questions raced through my frightened mind.

I lay on the operating table with my legs apart, propped up in stirrups. No sheet covered my naked body. While I was in this position, waiting for the operation to begin, I glanced around the room. It looked exactly like how I'd pictured the dirty, backroom abortion "clinics" I'd heard about during the days when abortion was illegal in the States, before *Roe v. Wade* was passed in 1973, the year before I joined the Peace Corps.

As I reviewed the unsterile conditions of the room, my eyes landed on a little kerosene camp stove with the instruments cooking in a pot on top. At that moment I became acutely aware of the risk I was taking. All the muscles tightened in my body as I felt dread pervade my insides.

The operation began with a few hostile comments on the part of the doctor, like, wasn't I "old enough to know better," and hadn't anyone taught me about birth control, followed by a few chuckles that made me shudder with anger. I lay on the table helpless, unable to properly defend myself verbally.

As the operation proceeded, the pain from the doctor forcing the instrument through my closed cervix and into my uterus became almost unbearable. The nurse held me down. I begged for some sort of anesthesia or numbing medicine. The so-called "doctor" said with a lurid smile that I didn't need any anesthesia. Amid my moans, he continued smiling and making hurtful comments like, "Now you will never forget this experience and you will be more careful next time."

I was so angry I yelled that I had changed my mind; I didn't want the abortion, and I wanted to go home.

The nurse gave me a tranquilizer to swallow with some sips of water. Of course, it didn't work right away. I felt no relief at that point. The pain from the instrument was unbearable.

While I moaned, the phone rang. The nurse handed the long-corded phone to the doctor as he sat between my legs, performing the abortion. I lifted my head to see what I would never forget.

With his left hand, the doctor held the receiver to his ear while the right hand scraped the inside of my uterus with a sharp instrument. I watched the large clock over my head. For five interminable minutes, the doctor laughed into the telephone amid my yelps of pain and pleas for anesthesia.

At nine o'clock, after I'd endured 35 minutes of physical and emotional torture and humiliation, the abortion was over. I bled profusely. The nurse gave me a Kotex pad and told me I could wait in the next room until the patient after me needed the room.

Holding the bloody pad between my legs, I hobbled to the cot, where I curled up, holding my still naked, aching belly. As soon as the nurse closed the door, I began to cry. My whole body trembled uncontrollably and my teeth chattered from the flood of adrenaline produced by the pain.

It seemed a long while before I regained control of myself. I decided I had to get out of this hateful place as soon as possible. I managed to get dressed. As I was leaving the room, I heard the screams of the next patient, screams that penetrated into my marrow. How many women must go through this torture? And how many women die or remain sterile the rest of their lives from infection?

This horrific experience left me feeling a deep sense of compassion for all the women throughout the world who have endured the terror and humiliation of backroom abortions. I made a pact with myself that whatever my purpose was in life, it had to include deep kindness and compassion—especially toward women.

The trip home on the crowded bus seemed endless. I bled heavily and began to feel lightheaded. At one point I nearly fainted, but I managed somehow to remain standing thanks to all the people pressed against me on the crowded bus. A woman saw what happened and gave me her seat.

I went to the house of Cindy, the kind friend who had helped me emotionally through the entire ordeal. I told her Ecuadorian parents that I was having an unusually severe menstrual period, and I asked if I could spend the weekend at their house with Cindy.

I spent the weekend in bed bleeding, drinking tea, and trying to regain my strength and self-respect.

I shared my tears and inner torment with Cindy. She asked me if I felt guilty about having an abortion. "I don't know if it's guilt I feel. It's more like sadness about having ended the little life inside of me. I pray that I'll have another chance to have a child when my circumstances are more stable. I want very much to be a mother someday."

Over time, I came to realize that I did indeed feel twinges of guilt. Even when I was a young child, it pained me to think that I might have caused harm to anybody—with a few exceptions. More recently, I had even felt a fleeting sense of remorse about using poison to kill the rats in my decrepit hacienda.

I hope I can forgive myself.

Monday I returned to language classes, but I still felt weak and continued to bleed. The bleeding persisted intermittently for two weeks.

Although I remained silent about what had happened, inner torment about the experience plagued me. Over time, I felt a compelling need to tell certain friends about the abortion experience.

The Peace Corps nurse found out about the abortion a few days later, when I went to her office to get checked. I wanted to see if the abortionist had done any permanent damage to my uterus. The nurse said I was incredibly fortunate not to end up with a serious pelvic infection.

After our appointment was over, the nurse handed me a year's supply of birth control pills. I put the little stack of boxes in my backpack, even though I could not imagine having sex with anyone for a very long time—maybe never.

Eventually someone informed the Peace Corps director about what had happened to me. A few weeks after my abortion, the Peace Corps newspaper published a short and inconspicuous article saying that the Peace Corps in Washington had just changed its policy concerning abortion, in keeping with the laws in the States. From that point forward, no Peace Corps volunteer would have to fear termination. The Peace Corps would pay for a round-trip ticket to the States for "medical reasons."

Long after I had recovered my emotional equilibrium, I wrote to Arthur about the accidental conception on the night of my departure. I gave him an abbreviated version of the abortion, leaving out the gory details.

Arthur wrote back several pages about his ambivalent feelings, wistfully pondering what it would have been like to raise a child together, but ultimately he felt relieved that I had an abortion. He had decided years ago not to have children.

In the letter, he said he wanted to travel to South America and rekindle our relationship. I wrote him back and told him about my relationship with Mateo. He decided to come anyway.

I suspected that the visit would not be a good idea, but I couldn't bring myself to tell him not to come. By trying to avoid hurting his feelings, I ended up indirectly creating more hurt. I still had a lot to learn about how to navigate relationships with men.

Chapter 24

LA COMPAÑÍA

ARTHUR HAD READ ALL the long and detailed letters I had sent to my parents, which they had shared with him. He wanted to see for himself what I had described. After spending a couple of days in Quito, he arrived in La Compañía. We had a heartfelt reunion with warm hugs.

Arthur confessed how surprised he was to discover that everything I wrote about in my letters appeared to be true, without any exaggeration. That unintentionally hurtful comment sounded familiar to me from my youth.

Even my own mother sometimes didn't believe me, like the time in my early teens I fainted in a medical museum in Washington, DC after looking at a huge disarticulated leg in a giant glass jar full of liquid. The former owner of the leg was an African man who suffered from a tropical disease called elephantiasis. As the blood left my head, I fell to the floor. Upon regaining consciousness, I looked up and saw a sea of faces staring down at me. I heard my mother say, "Don't pay any attention to her. She is just pretending she fainted."

Since I had gotten used to getting this kind of incredulous response to my behavior and stories throughout my life, I understood how Arthur might have made that assumption about what I wrote. If one has never traveled to remote areas, the kinds of experiences I've had would indeed seem beyond one's imagination.

Arthur and I never once mentioned the abortion during his visit. I sensed that he would not want to face the painful reality of my experience.

The people in the community thought that Arthur was my husband and had come to take me home—even though I'd told them multiple times that I didn't have a husband.

Pilar's husband, José, invited Arthur to join him for a hunting trip the day after he arrived. Arthur came back from the trip dizzy and exhausted. He spent the next day in his sleeping bag with symptoms consistent with altitude sickness, most likely due to his recent arrival at 12,000 feet above sea level. We had planned to climb a volcano with Mateo that weekend, but clearly we would need to cancel.

One of the men in the community had to travel to Quito for a work-related project. I gave him a slip of paper with Mateo's phone number and asked him to call Mateo from a pay phone in the post office. I told him to say that we couldn't go climbing together because my guest was sick, but he was welcome to come up to La Compañía to spend the weekend. I gave the man money to cover the cost of the phone call, plus dinner out for the trouble.

Seeing Arthur's distress from the altitude, I suggested we hike down the mountain and hang out at a restaurant in the town of Ambato. Arthur agreed.

In town, we ate a delicious breakfast of papaya, pineapple, banana, and a lemon, all chopped up together. We drank fresh-squeezed orange juice and hot chocolate. It felt good to come down from the mountain once in a while and soak in the amenities that the more developed places had to offer.

Arthur sat in his chair with a contented smile. All his symptoms had vanished.

We ran into another Peace Corps volunteer at the restaurant. She said she had two extra beds in the house where she stayed, and we were welcome to stay with her as long as we wanted. We spent the evening together sharing Peace Corps stories while listening to Carole King belt out her stirring songs on a cassette tape recorder.

The next morning, Arthur and I hiked back up the mountain. Upon our return, José gave Arthur one of the turtledoves he had shot and plucked. Arthur was repulsed by the thought of eating the little bird. Remembering the advice from my Peace Corps orientation, I ended up eating it myself, so as not to offend José.

The parents of the schoolchildren organized an outdoor celebration in honor of my "husband." The children gave a presentation of songs and contributed food they had cooked to the communal lunch. We helped ourselves to the corn on the cob and broad beans.

On one platter lay a boiled guinea pig, a delicacy that is typically served only on very important occasions, like weddings. One of the parents offered Arthur an arm with a little hand that still had claws attached. Arthur dry heaved, trying not to throw up. His being a strict vegetarian didn't help matters. When no one was looking, he fed the guinea pig arm to one of the dogs lurking around. I hoped no one had seen him do that; it would have been a human-relations disaster.

The people in these regions eat meat only about once a month because they cannot afford to eat it more often. Offering their precious guinea pig for this occasion was truly an honor.

The people seemed thrilled that I had a "husband." They treated Arthur with unrestrained generosity and warmth—quite a difference from the terrifying experiences I'd had when I first arrived in La Compañía.

During Arthur's visit, two of the local children invited Arthur and me for lunch in their home. Arthur said that the *chozas* were exactly as I'd described them in my letters to my parents. Arthur got to see firsthand what few outsiders ever see. He was in a state of awe most of the time.

On the second day of his visit, Arthur pulled from his backpack a beautiful Olympus camera that my parents bought for me. Finally I could ditch the Instamatic camera and take some good photos. Some of the people here had never seen a camera before I arrived with my Polaroid and little Instamatic. But over time they had become used to my camera and no longer ran away to hide.

Arthur decided to leave Ecuador only ten days into his planned three-week stay. He had a chronic headache from the altitude and struggled with a bad cold. But worse than that, he felt bummed out—more than a little—by my relationship with Mateo. When Mateo came up to La Compañía to visit me and to meet Arthur, the atmosphere became awkward among the three of us.

I felt sad when Arthur left. I could feel his disappointment. The visit had not turned out the way he had hoped.

> *I should have followed my instincts and told him not to come. I have trouble saying "No." I wonder if I'm trying too hard to be nice and not disappoint people. Men don't seem to have this problem.*

A few days after Arthur left Ecuador, the community had a festive gathering at the schoolhouse to mark the end of the school year. The schoolhouse, lent to the community by the *hacendado*, had one room for all the primary grades. The new school, with several rooms, would be finished by the time the children returned at the end of their summer vacation in late February.

All the parents appeared, loaded down with their colorful woven *shigra* bags containing fava beans, ears of corns, eggs, and bottles of *trago de caña*—a potent liquor made from fermented sugar cane. In addition to their heavy loads of food, mothers carried their babies on their backs, wrapped and secured with a shawl. The parents had come to bid farewell and offer their gifts of food and drink to Pilar, the community's beloved teacher. Pilar intended to return to her home, located an hour from La Compañía.

The activities included much drinking, speechmaking, and crying. The men offered alcoholic drinks with such insistence that I didn't dare refuse. I took a sip and then simply turned my face away and spit out the *trago*. The people were too drunk to notice. During these celebrations, the drinking often continued until loss of consciousness.

The headman, thoroughly intoxicated, offered his wife a *copa*—a small cup. She refused. "*Toma carajo!*" he shouted. ("Drink, damn it!") She drank obligingly, along with all the other women.

I thought the drinking orgy was on its last leg when I began walking back to the hacienda, but the crying and wailing began all over again. A dog joined in the howling. We all laughed as we wiped away our tears.

Pilar drove away with her husband into the setting sun like a hero in an old Western movie. The crowd dispersed and everyone stumbled home.

My parents requested in one of their letters that I write about a typical day. The day after Pilar's grand sendoff was a typical day for me.

At six-thirty in the morning I got up and answered the knocking in the doorway. It was the wife of the *huasicama,* the Indian who was the caregiver of the hacienda. This particular *huasicama* only had to take care of the *hacendado*'s animals since the hacienda was mostly in ruins, except for a few rooms in the main building where I lived. The woman had come to bring me my daily liter of fresh-squeezed goat milk, complete with twigs, hairs, and a few specks of dirt.

I got dressed and took my bucket to the irrigation ditch to haul water. I filled up the volcanic stone container that acted as a filter for the brackish water. The water dripped through the porous rock into an earthen jug below. I filled a big pot with this filtered water and put it on the stove to boil. In the meantime, I swept the floor and prepared breakfast with my homemade bread, boiled eggs, and the liter of goat's milk.

When the water boiled, I poured it into a basin and washed myself. Then I piled all the dirty dishes into a big container and lugged them up the hill to the irrigation ditch to wash them in the icy water. As I washed, I chatted with the people passing by. They gave me tips, like how to get pots to shine by scrubbing them with mud. One little boy asked me if Americans wear special dishwashing gloves in the water to keep their hands warm.

After finishing the dishes, I washed my clothes. An older girl asked me if it's true that Americans are so wealthy they don't even wash their dirty clothes—they simply buy new ones and throw away the dirty ones. I told the girl I had never met an American who did that.

As the people walked by, I greeted them with "*Imanala cangue?*" (Quechua for "How are you?") The reply was almost always the same: "*Aqui no mas, pasando la vida.*" (I'm simply here, passing through life.) The answer struck me as poetic, an expression of acceptance of their fate in life.

Rarely do the people here answer with whether they are fine or not fine. Maybe these concepts seem irrelevant to a person who is almost totally concerned with mere survival. Maybe they cannot afford the luxury of wondering if they are fine or not fine. Besides, this is their life—the only life they know.

I can't help thinking what a blessing it was that the people didn't have television sets to see how other people live—the people with lots of money and possessions. Envying other people could create another kind of misery.

Back at the hacienda I found my friend Alejandro waiting to give me my daily Quechua lesson. He was 12 years old and seemed to have a quick mind that grasps concepts easily. Along with some of the other students, Alejandro helped me work on the dictionary and transcribe legends. It was sometimes difficult to find a good source of information because often they just told you whatever they thought would please you. It could be frustrating.

During Arthur's visit to La Compañía, he met Alejandro. Arthur was so impressed with Alejandro's intelligence, he offered to give him a scholarship of 400 *sucres* ($15) a month for six years so he could go on to high school in Pujilí, almost five hours on foot from La Compañía. The parents turned down Arthur's generous offer, saying they didn't see the point of further schooling and that Alejandro was needed at home to help in the fields.

After my work session with Alejandro was over, it was already one in the afternoon. A little boy, Manuel, stood in the doorway, calling "Señorita Erica!" They used to call me *Patroncita*, which means "little boss lady." *Patrón* is a term used by the Indians when referring to white people. I told them I didn't want them to call me that. Gradually they dropped the deeply ingrained custom in my presence.

Little Manuel had come to bring me ten ears of corn and an invitation to lunch at his *choza*. We walked down the mountain together while he told me interesting information about our surroundings. He explained how he trapped the big bumblebees, how his family makes *chaur mishqui* (a sweet liquid that comes out of the middle of the agave cactus), how to tell the difference between the varieties of barley, and lots of other tidbits. On the way down the dirt path, we passed a young girl who said she had a legend to tell me. I told her to come to the hacienda in the afternoon to record it.

As we arrived at the *choza*, several members of Manuel's extended family were returning home after spending all morning working in the fields. The father offered me a little stump to sit on while everyone else either stood or squatted. The mother served me five ears of corn and 11 tiny boiled potatoes. For the second course we ate a watery soup with homemade barley noodles, onions, and potatoes.

After we ate, we sat for a few minutes while the food digested. One of the children was a four-year-old girl with delayed speech and only able to say a few words. She had grown accustomed to seeing me, since this was my third visit to her *choza*. When she saw me, she screeched with delight, "*Taita*," Quechua for "Daddy." After I finished eating, she crawled onto my lap and began fingering my earrings. She gave me a puzzled look and then reached for my breasts. She felt them through my thick wool sweater, and then, with a big smile of discovery, she announced, "*Mama*." I guess my blue jeans and my independence were enough to make me a man in her eyes—until she discovered otherwise.

Shortly after lunch, everyone dispersed to continue work in the fields. I went outside where one of the sons was threshing barley by beating it repeatedly with a long stick. He gave me a stick and we went at it together. After much beating, we fetched two pitchforks made of sticks tied together and began throwing the stalks into the air so that the wind would blow the chaff away and let the grain fall to the ground.

The men skillfully arranged the stalks into haystacks that looked like little round houses with conical roofs. The whole process made a very colorful scene. After a while, the son sat down with me and told me about all the damage the heavy and persistent rains had done. The grains had begun to rot with mold, causing general worry throughout the area.

On my way home, I stopped to pick a few young eucalyptus leaves, which I intended to put in my bed and rub on my body to keep away the fleas, lice, bedbugs, and other insects—a valuable tip I learned from the children.

As I neared the hacienda, I noticed that all my garbage had disappeared, except for the orange peels. There was no need to bury or burn my garbage here. The people picked it over and took home whatever could be of use to them. The dogs, pigs, and donkeys ate the rest. Needless to say, recycling was a natural part of life there.

When I arrived home, young Carmencita was waiting for me with her legend on the tip of her tongue. The story was short, containing a unique form of dry humor and involving a rabbit. Rabbits were often the villains or tricksters who outsmarted the innocent parties in a legend. She said, "A man had a store full of cheeses that he made every day. He began to notice that someone was stealing his cheese. He decided to hide and wait to see who it was. In came a rabbit to steal the cheese. The owner jumped out and grabbed the rabbit and said, 'Now I'm going to take you to jail.' The rabbit said calmly, 'Uncle, don't bother taking me all the way to jail. Let's just eat the cheese together.' So the owner and rabbit sat down together and ate up all the cheeses." Carmencita burst out laughing as though it was the most hilarious story in the world. Although I laughed too, I didn't really understand the meaning of the story, except that the rabbit outsmarted the man with the cheese. But I decided to include this story in the bilingual book anyway.

When evening came, it was time to light the candles and cook supper, relax, read, and fight off the cold and dampness that penetrates to the marrow. As I thought over the events of the day, I slowly faded into the world of sleep.

Thus ended a typical day in La Compañía.

One of the volunteers I ran into during a visit to the Peace Corps office told me a remarkable story that I never forgot. In her rural area, where she acted as an agricultural advisor, she had witnessed a huge measles outbreak within two neighboring villages. During that era, the World Health Organization, the WHO, had a stellar record for helping developing nations improve their public health by using some very simple, inexpensive measures—with much less reliance on astronomically expensive pharmaceutical drugs compared to current times.

The WHO dispatched health officials to the area of the measles outbreak and conducted a harmless experiment on the sick children. In the first village the children served as the control group for the study. Those children received no treatment for the measles except drops of water as a placebo. The second village served as the study group. Each sick child, including babies, received a huge dose of vitamin A drops once a day for about a week. The results showed a dramatic difference in the outcome in the two villages. Not a single child died in the group that received the short-term, high doses of vitamin A, and they had a remarkably quick recovery time, without any residual damage. The control group had three deaths and a much longer time to recovery.

Although I had no medical knowledge at that time, the fact that a mere vitamin could have such a dramatic healing effect never left my mind. In fact, vitamin A is part of my antiviral arsenal to this day. (High doses can only be taken for a few days and then must be stopped, or else the dose lowered to a more standard amount.)

The end of my two-year commitment in the Peace Corps loomed in the near horizon. The bilingual dictionary still needed a lot of work, but a couple of Peace Corps volunteers who worked in a village a few hours away said that they would ask for Pilar's help and continue to work on the dictionary until it was ready to be published and used in the local schools.

The bilingual book of folk legends lacked only some last-minute editing, which we got with the help of an older child who spoke Spanish quite well. Pilar had done most of the work already. One of the boys made a simple black-and-white drawing for the cover. Soon Pilar would take the book to Quito, where it would be published.

I dreaded the rapidly approaching day when I would have to say goodbye to my Ecuadorian friends, whom I had grown to love.

On my last day at La Compañía, all the people in the village came out to have a going-away party for *"La Señorita Erica."* As expected, someone handed me an entire roasted guinea pig impaled on a stick. I heartily ate the rodent and smacked my lips to show my gratitude. Several men handed me little cups of cane alcohol. I couldn't spit the contents out onto the ground without people noticing. I placed my hand on my stomach and made a vomiting gesture, at which point they stopped insisting that I drink with them.

A group of men sang in high-pitched voices, accompanied by home-made musical instruments, including a violin, guitar, panpipes, and something that looked like a mandolin. Tears rolled down my cheeks when I heard the mournful music, full of a sense of longing and mystery. I knew I was going to miss the Andes and these people whom I had grown so fond of.

Almost every person at the going-away party lined up to shake my hand and wish me well. I hugged all the children.

I got up at the first light of dawn the next morning and headed down the mountain with my heavy pack on my back that contained all my possessions. I sang a Quechua song that one of the children had taught me, trying to sing away my sadness.

By the time I reached the highway, my sadness began to lift. In its place came a rising sense of excitement as I anticipated meeting up with Mateo for our big climbing trip to Argentina.

Because Mateo had only a limited time to be away from the university for Christmas break, we needed to leave before I could say goodbye to my fellow volunteers. I would have to miss the Peace Corps goodbye party in January for the volunteers returning home to the States. I consoled myself, knowing I would surely remain in touch with a few of the volunteers whom I had befriended while in the Peace Corps.

Chapter 25

ACONCAGUA
THE ROOF OF THE AMERICAS

MATEO AND I, inseparable climbing companions, had talked endlessly about how we could make our dream of climbing Mt. Aconcagua a reality. Funding our own trip was not possible, given that Mateo was an impoverished university student and I made only $120 per month in the Peace Corps.

We decided to present our plans to the Sports Association of Quito and request funding from the Ecuadorian government. To our great surprise, the sports officials responded enthusiastically. They told us they wanted the Ecuadorian flag planted on the summit of Aconcagua, which would be a source of national pride. They offered to sponsor us on the condition that the trip would include at least four climbers, instead of just Mateo and me as we had originally planned. They wanted our trip to look like a true mountaineering expedition, not just two people on a "sentimental journey."

Mateo and I had wanted to climb Aconcagua alone, since these would be our last days spent together before I began my long, overland journey back home to the States. Grateful nevertheless to receive funding for our expedition, we complied with the Association's wishes and invited two more experienced climbers, Marcelo and Eloy, both from the climbing club called *Inti-Nan*. I had never met either of these men. Mateo had climbed with them only once. Fortunately, we all got along well together.

The Association gave us 10,000 *sucres* ($400) to cover expenses for the four of us. By South American standards in 1975, this was a large sum of money—yet not enough to permit us to travel by air, nor to stay in decent hotels.

Aconcagua, the Everest of the Andes, is located in Mendoza Province in Argentina, 15 kilometers from the Chilean border.

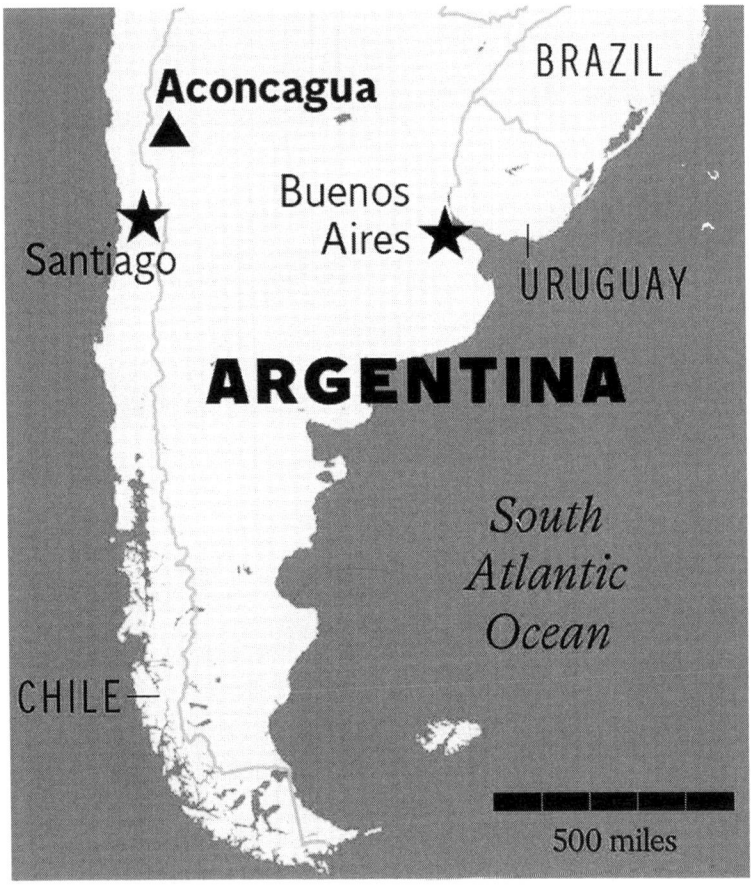

This towering mountain has lured climbers from all over the world for more than a century.

We planned our trip for December, which is midsummer south of the equator. That particular year had been designated by the United Nations as the International Year of the Woman, an auspicious time to make the climb. My climbing friends had done extensive reading about the history of climbing on Aconcagua. They told me that only seven women had reached the summit of Aconcagua. The first woman, Adrienne Bance from France, had reached the summit in 1940. They also told me that, as far as they knew, no American woman had made it all the way to the top, based on the list of entries in the ledger at the summit.

We left Quito on December 12. Aconcagua lay 5,695 kilometers and nine days of traveling away from Quito. We would spend close to a hundred hours on buses, with layovers in Lima and Arica in Peru, and in Santiago, Chile.

A rickety old bus with luggage and animals strapped on top took us through Ecuador. The bus was so crowded with people standing in the aisle that even turning around proved to be challenging. Marcelo had to sleep propped up in the aisle, sitting on the floor with all the other people without seats pressed against him. The smell of cigarette smoke, vomit, and stale urine from young children engulfed us.

The Chilean buses were much less cramped. When we finally arrived in Santiago, we decided to stay an extra day to rest and recuperate from our utterly exhausting travel. Mateo and I went to the beach at Viña del Mar, while the others explored the city.

The following morning at six-thirty, we caught the bus headed for the town of Mendoza, Argentina. All expeditions to Mt. Aconcagua must pass through there to get permission to climb the mountain.

When we finally got a clear view of the towering monolith with its vertical south wall, I felt a shiver of awe and fear run through my body.

Can I really do this?

As we bounced along the winding dirt road that took us up a steep mountain pass, I silently questioned whether I really wanted to go through with this climb. But the sheer anticipation and excitement overshadowed the doubts.

We found a cheap hotel in Mendoza. We could afford only one room with a single bed. Although the men offered to let me have the bed with a sagging mattress all to myself, I preferred sleeping on the wooden floor in my sleeping bag.

We spent three days in Mendoza, taking care of all the complex legalities involved in obtaining permission by the authorities to climb Mt. Aconcagua.

At police headquarters, we presented our packet of requisite documents. Besides our passports, the packet included letters of recommendation for each of us from the Sports Association of Ecuador, the lists of all the mountains each of us had ever climbed, and the years of experience we'd each had as climbers. Later, the police fingerprinted and photographed us.

Each climber had to pay a $10 refundable fee to cover the cost of removing his or her body off the mountain in case of death.

From there, the authorities directed us to the police doctor to see if he thought we were physically capable of attempting the climb.

The doctor hooked me up to various devices. The blood pressure monitor showed a reading of 95/50. The doctor said my low blood pressure showed that I was in good shape, but that if the pressure went any lower, I needed to take a heart stimulant called *Coramina*—which I never took. He said I would know my blood pressure was too low if I became lightheaded.

We had to run a few meters at top speed and then have our vital signs rechecked. The police doctor patted me on the back in a fatherly way and told me, "Congratulations! You are in unusually good health for a woman." I had become so used to sexism in South America that his words didn't faze me at all.

The police doctor asked me how I'd gotten so fit. I told him I had lived in a remote Indigenous Quechua community at 3,660 meters in the Ecuadorian Andes, where I spent much of my time recording, transcribing, and translating local legends into Spanish from the native Quechua language of the Inca descendants.

The police doctor became intrigued and wanted to know more about my life at high altitude in Ecuador. I briefly explained that life in the Quechua community was rigorous and primitive, without running water, electricity, latrines, stores, or clinics. The activities of daily living provided sufficient aerobic training for the massive volcanoes I climbed almost every weekend with my Ecuadorian friends in the climbing club.

He put his hand on my shoulder and said, "Then it's no wonder you are in such good shape. Perhaps your fitness will make up for your unimpressive gear." He smiled in a friendly way and then pronounced all of us physically fit. He sent us to get a psychiatric evaluation.

We could not find the psychiatrist. He had left for the day. After we gave the police doctor a small sum of money in exchange for his cooperation, he decided we showed no evidence of being mentally deranged or suicidal. He waived the psychiatric evaluation and signed the form, giving us the green light we needed to continue the approval process.

On the morning of our third day in Mendoza, the police ordered us to bring in all our equipment to be checked by the chief of security. This next hurdle worried us because our shoddy, mostly homemade equipment looked like it belonged to amateurs. Fortunately, I had my Kelty backpack, down jacket, and sleeping bag, which I had brought with me from the States.

A few professional-looking items lay among our pile of motley gear, like the barely-used Swiss climbing rope and two shiny metal ice axes with wooden shafts. Those pieces of high-quality gear were thanks to the times Mateo and I had guided European and American climbers in Ecuador. But our pile of equipment lacked some essential items, such as double boots to reduce the chance of frostbite, down pants, and bivouac gear for emergencies.

We held our breath as the police officer inspected our skimpy gear. He decided to overlook the glaring omissions because of our group's extensive mountaineering experience.

With a collective sigh of relief, we got the official stamp of approval on our final paperwork. We listened as the police official telegraphed an order to Puente de Inca, the army base that controls access to the mountains. The order gave us permission to climb Mt. Aconcagua. We let out yelps of relief and gave each other exuberant hugs.

We spent the rest of the day buying food supplies and over-the-counter medicines for our first aid kit, and then searching for a valve for the portable oxygen tank that we had borrowed from a hospital. We never found a valve that would fit our little tank; thus it was of no use. I felt anxious knowing that in case of an emergency, we would have no supplemental oxygen. My partners seemed relatively unconcerned by the idea.

That evening we each celebrated with a huge Argentine steak dinner that cost less than one dollar per plate.

On the morning of December 24, we caught the bus to Puente de Inca, an unusual army base at 8,800 feet, which looked more like a former ski resort with its massive stone buildings. The army base headquartered a training program for its mountaineer corps.

The name Puente de Inca, which means "Bridge of the Inca," refers to a natural bridge formed entirely out of yellow, brown, and white-colored mineral deposits left by the river that flows below the bridge.

Not far from the natural bridge, hot springs bubbled up from the ground. Bathhouses with huge stone tubs had been built into the rock. When an avalanche destroyed an adjacent hotel in the 1950s, the baths were abandoned and had since become covered with mineral deposits, creating an otherworldly appearance.

The officers at the army base gave us a hearty welcome and vigorously shook our hands. Once again, our equipment had to be checked, and once again we held our breath. The examining officer looked through our gear with a disapproving grimace. After discussing his concerns with us, he finally decided that since the police had approved of our gear, he would as well.

An officer told us to go to the infirmary for yet another physical examination to check our vital signs after we had jogged once around the grounds. The army doctor told us that the information he gathered on us and other climbers would be sent to the university in Buenos Aires, where scientists were studying the effects of high altitude on humans.

All of us had elevated red blood cell counts thanks to living at high altitude in Ecuador, where the oxygen pressure was significantly reduced.

We had seen many climbers who had not acclimatized to the altitude in the Andes develop acute "mountain sickness." The symptoms include headaches, nausea, vomiting, dizziness, irritability, apathy and, in extreme cases, loss of rational faculties.

Many of the expeditions to Aconcagua allow themselves up to a month on the mountain to acclimate. We allotted ourselves a total of ten days on the mountain, with the expectation that, since we lived at high altitude, we were already acclimatized and would not need much extra time.

Christmas Eve arrived just as we finished jumping through all the many hoops. We intended to begin our climb the next day, on Christmas.

We spent that evening soaking our bodies in the hot springs, and later into the night we drank delicious Argentine wine with the officers and soldiers. We all became gushingly sentimental and drank endless toasts to our families, friends, and each other.

On Christmas Day, the commanding officer informed us that our departure would be delayed until the following day due to the runoff from melting snows on the surrounding peaks. The muddy route had become impassable for the mules. The officer assigned a soldier to brief us about the mountain.

The soldier had obviously played this role many times and had all his facts in order. He said that a Swiss Alpine guide had reached the summit in 1897. The first woman to reach the summit was French, a member of an expedition that was led by a man called "Link" in 1940. The three-member party was killed as they were coming off the summit. It was rumored that Link had killed them and then killed himself in a moment of temporary psychosis from the altitude and extreme conditions.

We were told that more than 250 people had died on the mountain from various causes. A nearby cemetery housed the remains of some of those climbers. At the time of our expedition, eight dead bodies lay on the slopes of Aconcagua, including an American woman, Jeanette Johnson. The soldier said that her frozen corpse showed every indication of having been murdered. The story of her death remained in my thoughts. I wondered why no one had removed those eight corpses.

For the prior two years, Jeanette Johnson was a household name among climbers throughout South America, stirring the imagination and evoking feelings of mystery and fear.

Investigative journalists speculated about the possible motive for Jeanette's murder and also the murder of her fellow climber, John Cooper, a NASA official. Rumors ran wild and included the possibility that the CIA had planned the murder. The third member of the group, Zeller, was a policeman from Oregon. When Zeller came down off the mountain, officers at the army base asked about his partners. He stated that John Cooper had frozen to death and that Jeanette Johnson had disappeared.

The Argentine police contacted American officials and asked if they would like to have an investigation done. The officials declined the offer, so the case remained closed.

John Cooper's body was found shortly afterwards and taken down off the mountain. His skull was fractured and there was a wound where a presumed ice axe had penetrated his abdomen. When questioned about the findings, Zeller said they were caused by a fall. Yet, where Cooper's body was found, the grade was so minimal as to make a fall unlikely. Jeanette's body was nowhere to be found. The snows had covered all traces. The scene of this tragedy occurred at approximately 20,000 feet on the Polack Glacier.

The soldier's accounts of other strange deaths captured our imaginations. He told us about a Swiss couple who fought each other with their ice axes and later died, and a priest from Mexico who, upon reaching the summit, held out his crucifix, made a little speech about being close to God, and then flung himself off the edge.

Aconcagua appeared to have strange effects on some people's minds, due to the lack of oxygen and extreme fatigue. The soldier advised us to refrain from making jokes on our climb, since some people could be especially susceptible to irritability at high altitudes. An innocent joke, he said, could develop into a serious fight—even among the best of friends. At that point in the conversation, I wondered if I was making a mistake in attempting to climb this mountain. But then the thought of sharing this powerful experience with Mateo made me determined to go forward despite my fleeting moments of fear and doubt.

On December 26, we were ready for our departure. To cut down on the cost of gear-carrying mules, we decided to pack in everything ourselves on our backs, except for one 80-pound box of food. Two soldiers accompanied the mule we'd hired to transport our box of food. We agreed to meet the soldiers at the base camp on the third day, after the route had time to dry up.

We said goodbye to the comforts of the army base and to the many well-wishers who firmly shook our hands, gave us manly hugs, and stood watching and waving until we disappeared from view. Our grand send-off gave the impression that we were undertaking an important mission. Maybe we were. Or, maybe they thought we might not come back alive.

Chapter 26

GETTING CLOSE

The day was clear and crisp, and our spirits were high. We looked like pack mules with the loads on our backs. Mateo carried two full packs, one lashed to the other. The base camp for climbers lay 18 miles away—a two-day hike.

Soon after departing, we entered the narrow Valley of Horcones, named after a fork-tailed bird found in the region. The valley continued all the way to the base camp, called Plaza de Mulas, the place where the pack mules gather while the soldiers unload the supplies.

With Marcelo and Eloy walking ahead and out of earshot, I exuberantly expressed my love for Mateo. A man of few words, Mateo answered, "*Bebita, yo también te quiero tanto.*" Using a term of endearment, he said how much he loved me. He held my hand for a moment, pulled me gently toward him, and then we kissed briefly. From then on, the tone of the trip turned more serious.

By eight-thirty that morning, we arrived at Confluencias, where two rivers merge, the site of our first camp. After we set up our tents and rested for a few minutes, we walked around the area and found a tiny, cave-like construction made of rocks, obviously used as a shelter.

We arose at nine the next day, feeling no need to hurry. After hiking for two hours, we realized that we were east of our intended route and that the map the soldiers had given us showed misleading information.

From where the rivers merged, we had followed a neighboring canyon. After a loss of several hours, we regained our route near Piedra Grande, a large boulder where we stopped for lunch. The boulder marks the beginning of Playa Ancha, which means "Wide Beach," a rock-strewn channel about a quarter-mile wide and several miles long. In the late afternoon, the channel fills rapidly with water from the snows that melt in the midday sun, making a crossing treacherous.

Because we'd lost several hours in the morning, our timing was thrown off. We arrived at the far end of Playa Ancha just as the waters began to rush down like a flash flood. What was earlier a dry bed suddenly turned into an infinite number of snake-like streams that swelled rapidly. We hurried to reach the other side. We could easily jump over most of the streams or else throw in large rocks that served as stepping stones.

But before reaching high ground on the other side, we had to cross one last stream—one that had swollen to the size of a raging river. Mateo tied one end of the rope around his waist and managed, with great difficulty, to make it to the other side. Eloy, with his legs braced against a boulder, played out the rope from our side of the raging stream. Once on the other side Mateo belayed Eloy across, then threw the rope back to the other side so that I could rope up and then Marcelo. We precariously crossed the waist-high icy water, barefooted and barelegged, in our underwear.

We hiked until the light dimmed. We made camp without having reached base camp, which, we discovered the next day, was only 20 minutes beyond our campsite. With no water in our canteens and far from the streams, we camped in a state of dehydration. Before we crawled into our sleeping bags, we watched the moon as it filled the valley with its eerie light reflected off the glacier of El Cuerno, a peak directly before us. The spectacular sight helped to keep our minds off our dehydration.

We awoke to another sunny, cloudless day. We'd slept very little due to thirst, but the cold, invigorating air kept us moving at a brisk pace. We soon reached base camp, Plaza de Mulas, at 13,860 feet.

The camp's large shelter, a solid structure of wood and stone, looked like it could easily accommodate dozens of climbers. We tried the door, but someone had locked it. We discovered later that an expedition from Venezuela had locked the door on their way out and had taken the key, not realizing that we were due to arrive at that time. Fortunately, Mateo spotted an open window in the attic. He stood on Marcelo's shoulders and used his rock-climbing skills to hoist himself up to the little window and climb through into the attic.

The shelter looked like a palace to us, with its walls lined with provisions left by previous expeditions. If we'd known ahead of time about this abundance of food, we wouldn't have needed to hire a mule to carry our box of rations. On the other hand, it would be risky to count on always finding this kind of overstocking of food.

We soon understood why there was so much food left over from each expedition. The elevation and intense exertion often leads to loss of appetite. Most expeditions calculate the amount of food they will need based primarily on the number of calories they eat in their everyday lives. My normal consumption of around 3,000 calories per day shrank to less than 1,000 calories per day on the mountain. It seemed that digestion placed an additional strain on an already overtaxed system.

We spent the morning examining the contents of all the abandoned foods and medicines, trying to decipher the foreign words on the labels. Later we lounged in the sparse vegetation on the banks of the river behind the cabin. We rehydrated our bodies with cup after cup of delicious mountain-stream water.

Later that day, I prepared a package of dehydrated vegetable stew left by an American expedition. My three friends were pleasantly surprised and intrigued by the concoction, never having experienced a package of powder that instantly turns into a full meal.

In the late afternoon we heard a shout and rushed outside to greet two soldiers and the mule carrying our little-needed box of food. The soldiers lingered long enough to share our meal, then loaded up the extra equipment left by the Venezuelan party and began the long trip back to Puente de Inca with barely a moment of rest.

As evening approached, Mateo spotted in the distance two figures walking wearily toward the shelter. They were members of the Venezuelan expedition who had returned after reaching 18,000 feet, where exhaustion and *puna*—the local name for mountain sickness—had overcome them. The other two in the party had continued on toward the summit. We shared stories with the Venezuelans well into the night, so animated with excitement and anticipation that sleep was slow to come.

We arose at five the following morning, December 29. It was dark and cold when we left the shelter. After an hour, just as it was getting light, we passed another shelter, Plaza Vieja.

Along the way we noticed the carcasses of several dead mules in various states of decay. It was a gruesome sight. The soldiers had told us that the pack mules were dying of heart attacks. They explained that their hearts enlarged over time from the stress of working at high altitude.

Most of the day we silently zigzagged our way up a steep slope of fine, loose gravel. We put one foot in front of the other in a monotonous rhythm. The altitude made my heart race and pound like artillery fire. My mouth felt so dry, I couldn't resist a few big gulps from my canteen, in spite of warnings to sip water slowly. Immediately, I became nauseous.

Our rest stops were spaced at two-hour intervals, each being less than five minutes so we would not lose our pace.

At two that afternoon, we arrived at Antártida at 17,820 feet, a shelter that was only six-by-six feet and secured to the ground with heavy cables. Inside, we found the floor covered by a block of ice three feet deep. The flimsy door had been ripped open by high-velocity winds, allowing snow to enter, which had turned to ice.

We considered sleeping in our tents, but because of the slope's steep grade and the high winds, we decided to try our luck on the ice. We laid out a sheet of plastic and then piled all our possessions onto the plastic sheet, including ropes, ice axes, containers of food, and anything else that would serve as a buffer against the cold.

Before settling in for the night on my pile of equipment, I turned on my headlamp, took a pen from my pocket, and wrote on the plywood wall, "Erica Elliott was here with the Club Andino Politécnico de Quito, December 1975." Mine was only one of dozens of testaments written on the wall for posterity.

The night passed way too slowly. I moved around "in bed" constantly, trying to contend with the icy cold air and the objects poking into my back. But even worse than that, I had the dreaded *puna*. The pain in my head became intense, worse than a migraine headache. I finally gave in and let Mateo inject me with Darvon. This allowed me to sleep one half-hour before it was time to get up.

At the first signs of light, we stumbled out of the shelter, looking haggard. In a daze from the pain medication and from lack of sleep,

I made coffee for us and shared a few of my snacks. The men were restless to get going. We packed up our gear and continued up the mountain. I wondered how I could possibly make it to the summit, but kept my thoughts to myself.

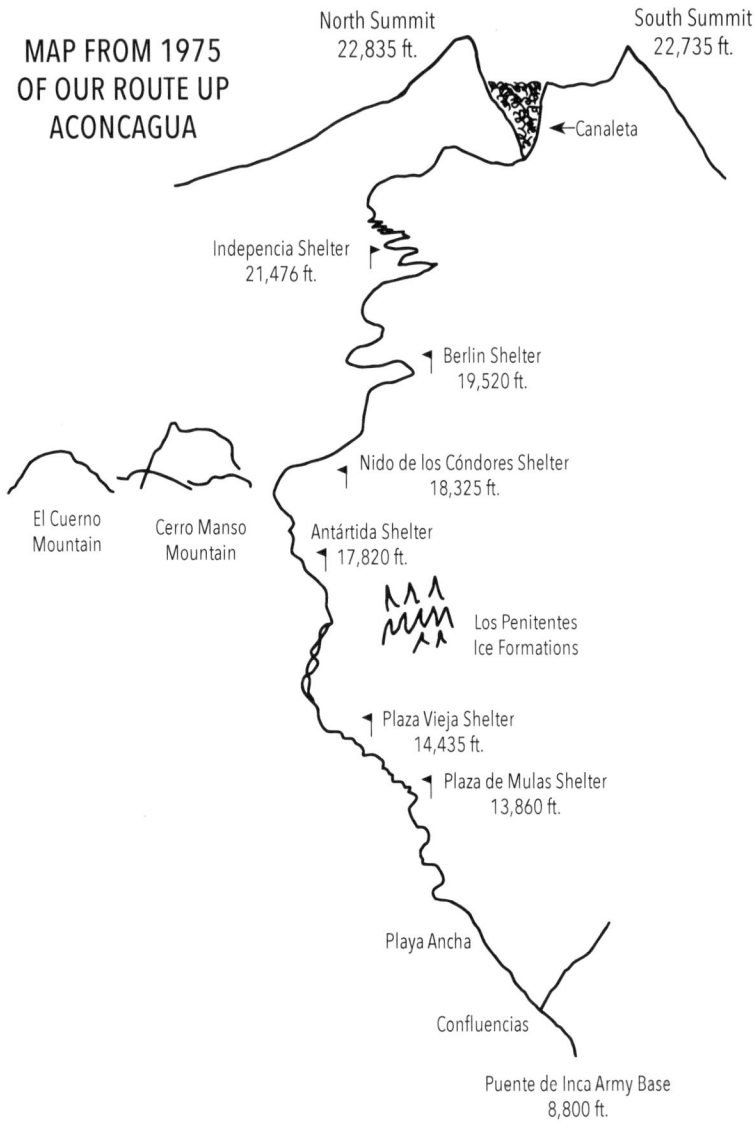

After two hours of putting one foot in front of the other, and after passing Nido de los Cóndores (Nest of the Condors), we arrived at three little shelters located at approximately 20,000 feet. The first two miniature A-frames were not habitable due to the ice inside, which had accumulated to the top of the little doors, making entry impossible. The third shelter, called "Berlin" in honor of the German scientists who had donated it, was accessible and a bit larger than the other two, allowing space to stand up. Cables held down the shelters so that they could withstand the powerful winds that came sweeping down off the summit.

In Berlin we took off our heavy packs, rested for a half-hour, and then pushed on. After 45 minutes, we met the other half of the Venezuelan expedition coming down from the summit. They said they had made it to the top. Yet when we asked them about it, their claims sounded dubious, since they hadn't seen the aluminum cross nor the summit book—both of which were in plain sight upon reaching the top, according to the soldier who oriented us at the army base.

The soldier at Puente de Inca had told us it was not uncommon for climbers to say they had reached the summit when in fact they had not. They could prove their success by signing the summit book, taking photos, or bringing back souvenirs left by previous expeditions—swapped for their own objects left behind—a custom found throughout the Andes.

In any case, the Venezuelans cautioned us to return to the Berlin shelter to get an early start the following morning. According to them, the summit lay ten hours away.

Taking their advice, Mateo, Marcelo, and Eloy accompanied the Venezuelans down as far as Antártida, where they gathered the rest of our equipment that we had left, having mistakenly thought that we could make the summit and back to Antártida in a day.

I stayed in Berlin melting pan after pan of snow for soup and tea. When my chores were over, I went to a rocky overlook to watch the progression of my friends as they wound their way back up the side of the mountain. I noticed that Eloy's pace had become unusually slow. He rested every few steps in a sitting or lying down position. When he approached I saw how sick he looked, but he insisted that he was feeling all right.

We did little the rest of the afternoon besides preparing our equipment for the following day. By eight o'clock we were in our sleeping bags, but none of us slept. It was probably the most miserable night of my life. There was little oxygen. We had to consciously monitor our breathing so that our lungs would keep expanding to their full capacity. The air was stuffy, with no ventilation. In desperation I slept with my nose in the slightly opened door.

Mateo asked me to close the door because Eloy had developed a fever and a hacking cough. On top of that, I had developed a full-fledged case of *puna*. I had to remain in a sitting position the entire night. Lying down brought excruciating pain to my head. Mateo again injected me with Darvon, but it brought no relief this time.

We were all dehydrated because the water in our canteens had frozen. The temperature was ten degrees Fahrenheit inside the shelter. We had to get up in the middle of the night to melt snow for tea. I noticed that getting up and moving around brought some relief.

Mateo's little alarm clock rang at three in the morning on the last day of the year. Our spirits were low and our minds foggy. Eloy's condition had become serious. He was gasping for air and alternating between sweating and freezing from the fever. We plied him with hot tea all through the night, along with a dose of the antibiotics we had bought at the drugstore in Mendoza. We waited for the morning to come so that someone could take Eloy off the mountain before he got too sick to walk.

Now came the problem: Who was going to take Eloy down? I felt that we should all stay together as a group. Marcelo replied that this was their only chance to try to make the summit, since they had to be back in Quito for the start of classes. When someone suggested that we forget about attempting the summit, Mateo said he felt he owed it to the Sports Association, since they had paid for our trip.

After more discussion, Mateo offered to accompany Eloy down off the mountain himself. Everyone voted against that idea because he was the team leader. Marcelo said that I should be the one to go down since I had the worst case of *puna*. We all became irritable and argumentative. I could feel myself slipping into sleep-deprived and pain-induced irrationality. The tears streamed from my face as I told of my dreams of climbing to the summit with Mateo.

"And today is the last day of the International Year of the Woman," I babbled, my behavior convincing them all the more that I should be the one to go down with Eloy.

In a flash, I came to my senses as I took in the absurd scene unfolding, with the three of us huddled around the burning candle, arguing about who should take Eloy down, while Eloy sat in the corner gasping for air. In a moment of clear thinking, I agreed that I should be the one to take Eloy off the mountain.

Marcelo and Mateo hastily prepared for their departure to the summit. By six-thirty, they were on their way up the mountain, as Eloy and I headed down. They later filled us in on what happened.

They reached the summit in five hours, breaking all previous records, pushing themselves at an inhumane pace so that they could beat the bad weather that was brewing. A mushroom-shaped cloud had engulfed the entire summit, which meant the "white wind" would soon follow, a blinding wind made of particles of snow and ice. They were frightened. Their feet had become frozen, like lifeless stumps. At one point, they stopped, took off their boots, and massaged each other's feet until the circulation returned.

Marcelo had difficulty breathing and had episodic hallucinations involving crosses. He tried to convince Mateo that they had reached the summit because he knew there was supposed to be a cross on top. He began to photograph the crosses, which were just thin air, a projection of his weary, oxygen-starved mind.

When they finally reached the true summit, Marcelo got down on his hands and knees and began throwing rocks around as though he were looking for something. When Mateo asked him what he was doing, he said he was looking for the shingles on the "roof of America."

By two in the afternoon they were back in Berlin, where they waited out a snowstorm.

In the meantime, after an exhausting six-hour descent, I managed to get Eloy down to Plaza de Mulas, where a Japanese expedition had just arrived. Communicating with them was comical. They spoke only a few words of English and Spanish. A doctor on their expedition managed to convey to us that Eloy probably had bronchitis, complicated by pulmonary edema. The drop in altitude had significantly alleviated his difficulty breathing, yet he still needed medical help to prevent pneumonia.

After entrusting Eloy to the care of the attentive Japanese doctor, I spent the rest of the day sitting by the river, trying to sort out my jumbled feelings. The tears rolled down my cheeks. I had succumbed to the stresses of the many sleepless nights we had endured from the time we left Quito two weeks earlier.

After one restful night, I recovered my emotional equilibrium. It took a little longer to let go of the disappointment I felt about not being able to climb to the summit with Mateo. But I was also relieved that Eloy got down the mountain safely and was out of imminent danger.

That evening Mateo and Marcelo staggered into Plaza de Mulas looking like wild men in a stupor. Their faces were swollen and disfigured, a frightening sight. They were too exhausted to talk.

The moment I saw them, I realized how fortunate I was that I agreed to take Eloy down the mountain. I could have never made it to the summit in the condition I was in.

The next day, a soldier packed Eloy out on a mule. It was New Year's Day, a fact we didn't even talk about.

After a few hours of rest, Mateo, Marcelo, and I began the long hike back to Puente de Inca. We walked without talking to each other. Mateo and Marcelo's pace had become uncharacteristically slow from exhaustion. We stopped at Confluencia and spent the night in a cave, too tired to set up our tents. Mateo and Marcelo slept until three o'clock the following afternoon.

On the way to Puente de Inca the next day, we passed the carcass of a mule. With a shudder, I recognized the white markings on its face, identifying him as the one who had carried up our box of food. His swollen body had burst open, allowing his entrails to spill out. He had died presumably from a heart attack. A wave of horror and sadness passed over me.

As we were leaving the Valley of Horcones, we met two Argentine priests camped by the lake. They were spending two weeks acclimatizing in preparation for their third attempt to climb Aconcagua. When I mentioned my disappointment about not making it to the summit, they agreed to let me climb with them. I told them that if I decided to come back, I would join them in a few days.

At Puente de Inca, the soldier who oriented us gave Mateo and Marcelo a heartfelt congratulatory handshake. A climber had relayed the news of their extraordinarily rapid ascent to the summit. Later we found Eloy recovering under the care of the army doctor.

We showered, went for a brief medical examination, and then headed to bed. Marcelo and Mateo slept for 15 hours. I got into bed with Mateo and put my arm around him while he slept. Waves of sadness made my heart ache as my mind wandered to our imminent separation. The thought was almost unbearable.

I spent the next afternoon watching soldiers stop every passing vehicle to check for suspected terrorists, concealed weapons, and ammunition. Argentina's continual political upheavals had grown more intense now due to the severe inflation that racked the country.

On the morning of our departure from the army base, after Eloy had fully recovered from his episode of pulmonary edema, one of the soldiers flagged down a passing car and ordered the driver to take all four of us to Mendoza. We spent the day in the city running errands and resting up for the next leg of our trip. For Mateo, Marcelo, and Eloy, the next leg meant another 100-hour bus trip back to Ecuador.

One evening in Mendoza, as we sat quietly eating dinner in a cheap restaurant, total chaos suddenly broke out when five policemen kicked open the door, marched in with guns drawn, and ordered everyone to go to the wall with their hands over their heads. I barely breathed, waiting to get shot in the head as I stared at the wall in front of my face. I wondered if my parents would be notified of my death. I wanted desperately to tell my mother and father that I loved them before I died.

The police inspected each person's identification papers, then patted us down. They hit some of the men and shoved them, telling them to line up at the door. The police took those men somewhere—probably to jail or worse.

We sat back down at our table in an adrenaline-soaked daze. The waiter said this sort of occurrence was so common that it didn't even reach the newspapers.

When we left Mendoza, we took the bus to Santiago, Chile, the place where I tearfully parted ways with my companions. We gave each other long, heartfelt hugs.

I told Mateo I would write him lots of letters while I traveled, and that we would see each other again in a few months when I passed through Quito on my way home. With a choked-up voice, I told Mateo how much I loved him and that I would keep a place for him in my heart for the rest of my life. Mateo looked down at the floor so no one would see him crying.

While my friends headed back to Quito to resume their classes at the Polytechnic Institute, I stayed in Santiago a few days to plan my trip around the continent for the next six months before returning home.

Before leaving Quito, I had cashed in my $600 return ticket to the States on Pan American Airways, enough money to last for about six months while traveling in South America.

I wandered around Santiago aimlessly, heartbroken about leaving Mateo and intensely missing my climbing companions, not able to hold back my tears. We had shared several years' worth of experiences compressed into a few weeks. I seriously pondered the possibility of returning to Ecuador and spending the rest of my life with Mateo. My rational mind talked me out of pursuing that path. I wondered, though, if Mateo would ever consider moving to the States to live with me.

That night, if I had any liking for alcohol, I would have gotten drunk. Instead, I fully experienced the pain. When I saw lovers walking hand in hand down the street, or stopping to kiss and hug each other, I had to wipe away my tears and swallow hard.

After several days of coming to grips with my aching sense of loss, I decided to change my plans and postpone for a couple of weeks my trip around the continent. I felt a magnetic pull to return to Mt. Aconcagua and join the priests. I wanted to reach the summit as an expression of my love for Mateo and the dream we had.

Chapter 27

THE RETURN

EARLY ON THE MORNING OF JANUARY 11TH, I caught a taxi out of Santiago. It broke down after a few miles. I got out and within minutes a VW van stopped. A Uruguayan family traveling all over Latin America in their van, American-style, invited me to ride with them. We had a delightful time laughing and sharing stories of our adventures. Without my asking, they drove me to Puente de Inca—far out of their way.

During the ride, the mother asked why it was so important to me to make it to the top of Aconcagua. I explained that climbing was a spiritual endeavor that had taught me important life lessons. She asked me what exactly were those life lessons. I struggled to express the answers clearly.

I told her that I had learned to be brave and practice good judgment when facing danger, and not make rash decisions based on fear. And I learned that I was capable of far more than I ever realized. I also learned that, against all odds, by simply putting one foot in front of the other and not giving up, I would eventually reach my goal—in this case, the goal would be the summit.

The mother responded, "Ah, the mountain is a metaphor for you." Yes, it certainly was.

I shared with her the Navajo grandmother's prophecy after my close encounter with the mountain lion. The grandmother said that I needed to make myself strong in mind and body for what lay ahead. She said that I would face some life-threatening obstacles. I forgot the rest of the prophecy, which I had written in my diary, stored at my parents' house in New Hampshire.

That tiny glimpse of my history piqued the family's curiosity, but we had to end the conversation because we had arrived at the army base.

I wished I could have continued traveling with the delightful Uruguayan family. While talking and laughing with them in their van, I temporarily forgot how much I longed to be with my tribe of Ecuadorian friends—especially Mateo.

The major at the army base informed me that the priests were already on the mountain, having assumed I wouldn't return. The major forbade me to climb alone, so I resigned myself to waiting for another expedition to arrive. He asked me to give him my word.

Without my Ecuadorian climbing companions, the atmosphere of the army base was less inviting with its macho, women-hungry soldiers to cope with.

By a stroke of luck, an Argentine expedition from Buenos Aires arrived, led by a 61-year-old man whom I will call Tomás, a well-known climber in Argentina with a reputation as a diehard. He had led seven expeditions to Aconcagua, three of which had made it to the summit. His 18-year-old son, Alberto, and two friends—Raúl in his late twenties, and Carlos in his early thirties—accompanied Tomás. The press had given much publicity to his expedition. The officers at Puente de Inca treated Tomás like a VIP, giving him free room and board, all of which made me suspect he had connections with one of the commanding officers.

I told Tomás the story of my time on the mountain and requested permission to join his group. He initially expressed doubts about having a woman on his team, but after I presented my credentials, he enthusiastically welcomed me aboard.

After being ordered to run one kilometer, we had to submit to a physical examination similar to the one I had received with my Ecuadorian friends. The doctor said I had a set of lungs "like a horse" and that my red blood cell count had increased by about one million since my last checkup. I was pleased knowing that now my body had become even more acclimated, which would make this expedition less grueling.

In the evening, one officer and his wife invited us to their home for champagne and dessert. He told us that the Japanese expedition had reached as far as the hut called "Independencia" at 21,000 feet, but they had to turn back because of a snowstorm. During my time in Santiago the weather on Aconcagua had become stormy, making access to the summit difficult.

After his wife excused herself to go to bed, the officer regaled us with his storehouse of information about Mt. Aconcagua, including vivid tales of tragedies that had occurred on the mountain. With difficulty, we pulled ourselves away for bed.

As we were leaving, the officer took me aside and whispered that he would like to meet me later. When I said that I wasn't interested, he countered with, "I thought all American girls like a little fun." He reached for my breasts. I removed his hands off my body. As I walked out the door, I said, "That's no way to treat a woman. What would your wife say about your behavior?"

We finally got under way at eleven-thirty the next morning. I felt happy, full of energy and anticipation.

After walking a few hours, the four men began slowing down and showing signs of fatigue and shortness of breath. They had to take frequent rest stops. They lived in Buenos Aires at sea level and weren't acclimatized.

I offered to carry Tomás' 55-pound pack the rest of the way while he carried mine, which was considerably lighter. At first he declined my offer, no doubt embarrassed by the prospect of a woman carrying the heaviest load, but eventually he accepted gratefully. It made me happy to contribute something to this party that was so generous in letting me join them and partake of their food and company.

In the late afternoon we passed two people on mules. The soldier on the first mule led a second mule that carried a Mexican climber sick with pneumonia. The sick man looked flushed with fever and appeared delirious. The soldier stopped briefly to tell us what happened.

The Mexican was with his compatriots in Antártida when he suddenly became ill with a high fever and a hacking cough. A member of the expedition rushed down the mountain to get help. Fortunately, he found a soldier in Plaza de Mulas, who set out at once, ill equipped for such an unforeseen undertaking.

In record-breaking time, the soldier climbed to Antártida—a feat in itself—and then carried the tall, 200-pound Mexican down the mountain in the middle of the night. He slid his body, bundled in a sleeping bag, over the snow and ice, but often he had to drape the body over his back when the terrain was rough. When he encountered smooth terrain, he dragged the body. They arrived back at Plaza de Mulas at five in the morning. The soldier had worked nonstop for 20 hours to save the Mexican man's life. Now they had to wait for the next mule to appear to transport the sick man back to the army base.

I woke everyone up at 5:45 the next morning with the intention of getting under way early to avoid the hazardous crossings of the rivers, which swell in the late afternoon at the end of Playa Ancha. Only after I had washed the dishes from dinner the night before, fetched water, made breakfast, and begun packing up my equipment did the group manage to crawl out of their sleeping bags. I wondered if the altitude had already begun affecting them.

At noon, just as we were entering Playa Ancha, a tremendous wind came roaring down through the valley with a force that continued for several hours, sending the soil airborne. Our bodies were covered with dirt; we looked like children who had played in the mud all day. We walked with our heads bent low and sometimes could not walk at all. I tasted the dirt in my mouth. My eyes stung. I reminded myself that the wind served as a blessing in disguise. It meant that the temperature was very cold high on the mountain, preventing the snows from melting and the rivers from rising and becoming impassable for us.

In this barren landscape, we saw few animals aside from rabbits, hawks, and eagles. As I walked, I heard a low, trumpet-like call from above. Tomás said that it was a male guanaco, an animal related to the llama but smaller. His call warned his harem that we were approaching.

We arrived at another small, cave-like shelter named "Ibañez" after the first and most famous Argentine climber. Carlos and Alberto did not want to go any further. Carlos said his legs ached and Alberto complained of blisters on his feet. We agreed that the two of them would camp in the cave for the night while the rest of us kept walking. They planned to catch up with Raúl, Tomás, and me at Plaza de Mulas the next day.

The next morning, as we hiked to Plaza de Mulas, Tomás threw up his breakfast along the way. I asked if he wanted to stop and rest.

"I'm fine. Stop worrying about me," he answered, obviously embarrassed about his condition.

At Plaza de Mulas, about six different expeditions filled the large shelter that served as the base camp. We saw eight Swiss mountaineers asleep on the floor on their mats. One of the Swiss men said that the high level of freshly fallen snow had prevented them from reaching the summit. A British climber said he couldn't get beyond Antártida due to the bad weather.

A group of ex-soldiers, formerly stationed at Puente de Inca, had chosen Plaza de Mulas for their annual reunion. Tomás said that each of the ex-soldiers had extensive experience as skiers and mountaineers and had participated in many rescue operations, bringing climbers off the mountain dead or alive. With them was a man of German origin, Willy Noll, who caught my attention because of his demeanor as a natural leader.

It was late before our excited conversations subdued and we crawled into our sleeping bags.

We waited all the next day for the mules to bring up our food supplies. We passed the time getting to know each other, taking pictures, greasing our boots to waterproof them, exploring the surroundings, and sunning ourselves. We listened to the soldiers brag about their exploits on and off the mountain. All from elite, upper-class families, they had served their obligatory time in the army. They were friendly and kind, but their machismo behavior sometimes grated on my North American sensibilities.

By evening the mules still had not arrived. Raúl, Tomás, and I decided to leave for Plaza Vieja, a one-hour hike above us. There is a steep hill called "La Questa Brava"—The Terrible Hill—not far from the shelter. It is normally a 20-minute hard climb. When I reached the top, I saw a group of soldiers below cheering and waving. They had timed me in their competitive spirit. I had reached the crest in nine minutes with a full pack. They nicknamed me "La Cabra Montés"—the mountain goat—a nickname that stuck throughout the rest of my time on the mountain.

When we reached the little shelter, we received a warm welcome from the two priests I had met earlier, along with two other members of their party. They'd been delayed by weather on the upper part of the mountain, which allowed us to catch up to them. The shelter felt cozy, located near a stretch of unique and dazzling ice formations called "Los Penitentes."

The priests left the next morning for the shelter Antártida. I felt torn between going with the priests, who were more acclimatized and had a faster pace, and staying with Tomás and his group, who were not well acclimatized. After much reflection, I decided to stay with Tomás' group because I was well acclimatized and could offer them moral support and encouragement, as well as help them with the chores and with their heavy packs.

Raúl, Tomás, and I spent the morning exploring and climbing around in Los Penitentes, ice formations that look like huge towers. Tomás said that only Aconcagua and the Himalayas have such ice formations.

At noon Carlos and Alberto, still tired and weak, finally joined us. They reported that the mules had arrived with our provisions. Three of us went down to Plaza de Mulas to fetch part of our food.

The ex-soldiers climbed to Plaza Vieja and camped in their tents beside the shelter. Through binoculars, we saw that the route to the top was improving as the snows melted from the bright sunlight.

Our group had a slow, labored pace when we left the next morning. Sometimes I waited half an hour for the others to catch up. My body became chilled while I waited. Soft, mushy snow lay on the ground. Our boots got wet despite all the greasy treatments we had carefully given to the leather. The men were discouraged; I tried to raise their spirits. The three youngest men agreed that this was the hardest thing they had ever done in their lives. Little did they know what still lay in store for them.

After 11 long hours of struggle, they finally arrived at Antártida with their last gram of strength. Carlos arrived at the shelter without his pack. He said he couldn't go on with it, so he left it a few hundred feet below the shelter. I retraced my steps and retrieved his pack. When I arrived back at the shelter, Alberto and Carlos were arguing heatedly. Alberto was apparently angry at Carlos for his strange behavior. They were both victims of altitude and fatigue. Alberto had become irritable and Carlos irrational—symptoms I knew all too well from the previous expedition, although this time it had struck at a much lower altitude.

I realized that the group would have to spend at least a day acclimating themselves before they could continue. I decided to continue my climb up to Berlin to join the priests, and then rejoin Tomás again in a day. But I was not gone for more than a couple of hours before I realized I could not make Berlin before midnight. I repeatedly sank to my knees in the wet snow. I turned back.

The moon was full, illuminating the snow and casting strange shadows. It was a comforting feeling to get back to my friends in the matchbox, six-by-six shelter. The ice remained inside, but this time we had better insulation pads. Our major problem was how to fit all five of us in this tiny space. Four of us lay lined up on our sides while Alberto lay across the pads just below our feet.

I offered to prepare dinner, but no one was hungry. They had eaten nothing all day except for a light breakfast. They drank some liquids and then went to sleep. We passed the canteen around at intervals

The Return

all through the night to fight off dehydration. I heard Alberto moaning from the pains in his head.

Tomás awoke with a burning sensation in his eyes. He had lost his vision. He had gone without his goggles for about an hour the day before, enough time for the reflection of the sun off the snow to burn his corneas. He spent the day in his sleeping bag with his eyes bandaged.

All four of Tomás' group suffered from *puna*, with excruciating headaches. Medicines offered no help. Carlos feared that his head would literally split open. He packed his belongings and said he was going home. He left without saying goodbye. I felt sad to see him go, but also relieved to know that his physical suffering would soon be over.

The other three spent the entire day in their sleeping bags trying to sleep. Persistent nausea prevented them from eating. In the afternoon I went off by myself to climb a neighboring peak, Cerro Manso. It was an easy climb with a magnificent view at the top. In the thin air, I could see all the way to Plaza de Mulas.

Tomás, Raúl, and Alberto all felt wretched the next morning with *puna*. Thankfully, Tomás' vision had returned. At noon the Argentine priests stopped by on their way down the mountain. They had gotten as far as Independencia at 21,000 feet before exhaustion stopped them.

In the afternoon we left Antártida. Soft snow and mud still covered the route, making walking tedious and slow. After four and a half hours, we arrived at Berlin. The men were panting and bleary-eyed.

In Berlin, while waiting for the others, I spoke with the Mexican climbers whose friend had been evacuated due to pneumonia. The beer company where they worked in Mexico City had sponsored their trip—all expenses paid, including a trip to the States to buy their equipment at REI in Seattle. Why? So they could get a photo of the company flag flown from the highest piece of land in the Americas.

The group finally made it to the summit after a 14-hour struggle. Rosa Maria, the first Mexican woman ever to reach the summit, had become barely able to function during the last five hours of the climb due to profound exhaustion. They had already been off the summit for a day, yet the altitude still showed its effects. Their bodies looked swollen, most noticeably in the face and hands, and their skin had a grayish hue. Their speech was unclear, and they had a look of apathy. They had spent six days at this altitude. The army doctor told me that brain cells begin to die after a prolonged period at high altitude, and this can result in permanent brain damage. I was relieved to hear that they planned to descend the mountain the following day.

I spent most of the day walking around, melting snow, writing in my diary, and preparing for the ascent the next day. It's normal at this altitude to accomplish very little in a day because everything must be done in slow motion so as not to waste any energy and overextend oneself.

In the evening, in a moment of relief from his headache, I asked Tomás to tell me the story about how he had discovered Jeanette Johnson's corpse. A year after she had disappeared, Tomás climbed the Polack Glacier with a party from Buenos Aires. At about 20,000 feet, not far to the east from where we had been climbing, Tomás spotted something in the snow. He hiked over to the object and found a perfectly preserved corpse of a woman. Tomás immediately assumed the body was that of Jeanette Johnson. The skin on her face had blackened and her eyes were burned out from the sun.

Tomás removed her ring to present to the police as proof of his story. He piled up rocks to mark the spot in case the snows should once again entomb her body. She had frozen into a solid block of ice. In 1976 a team of soldiers finally brought her body down the mountain and shipped it back to the States.

Weeks later, when I visited Tomás at his home near Buenos Aires, I saw the gruesome slides he had taken of her corpse to show to the police. Her face looked twisted, her mouth open in an expression of terror. She was entangled in her rope and her body and face were bruised.

Tomás also told me about a time, a few years before, when he'd found a boot with a foot in it, not far from Independencia. No one at the army base had any explanation for the grim discovery. I wondered if an animal had eaten the rest of the body.

Tomás' headache finally subsided enough for him to fall asleep. The next morning, he noted that he had an abnormally low heart rate, considering the altitude. He felt lightheaded and feared that low blood pressure was causing his symptoms. I made up a quart of tea for him to drink and gave him my bottle of *Coramina*, the heart medicine that the army doctor had given me in case my heart rate and blood pressure dropped below normal.

When I saw no improvement in Tomás, I told Alberto and Raúl to take him down off the mountain. Another climber heading down the mountain agreed to accompany the three of them all the way to Plaza de Mulas. We gave each other heartfelt hugs. I thanked them for having allowed me to join their group and said I would visit them in Buenos Aires.

Chapter 28

THE VIEW FROM THE TOP

WHILE CAMPING IN MY TENT not far from the Berlin shelter, I encountered two brothers, ex-soldiers I had met during their reunion at Plaza de Mulas. I will call them Santiago and Rodrigo for the sake of anonymity, given their current positions as officials in the Argentine government.

I saw the brothers hastily preparing their gear for an ascent to the summit the following morning. I asked if I could accompany them. Without hesitation they denied my request. They felt certain that a woman would slow them down and prevent them from reaching the summit.

I convinced them that if this should be the case, I would turn around and head back to Berlin by myself while they continued on. I also pointed out that I had equipment they might need, like an ice axe, slings, and a pair of crampons. They reluctantly agreed to let me follow behind them.

Before six the next morning Santiago, Rodrigo, and I left Berlin and headed up the mountain with only hot tea in our stomachs. We walked in the dark, with a cold wind in our face.

Santiago and Rodrigo began walking at a rapid pace. I suspected they were trying to show that I couldn't keep up with them. I knew it wouldn't be long before they wore themselves out.

We had only been climbing for an hour when Rodrigo asked if I could carry the one pack we had for the three of us. I willingly agreed.

We arrived at Independencia (21,000 feet) in less than two hours. Independencia was another tiny, A-frame shelter that was used only in emergencies. It had a large hole in the roof, over a foot in diameter.

My feet began to freeze. I had on two pairs of wool socks to make up for not having double boots, which would have been more appropriate. I tried to move my toes. My feet began to feel like stumps beneath me. Fears of frostbite and amputation filled my mind. I calmed myself with the realization that the sun would appear in a matter of minutes.

After two hours of walking, we encountered extensive snow and ice on the route, much more than we expected. The brothers lacked proper equipment for snow and ice, having only ski poles.

This particular route, referred to as the "normal route," usually offered little in the way of snow and ice climbing, the challenge being more about physical and mental endurance than technical skill.

Not far above Independencia, we came to the Shiller Glacier, named after a geologist who had frozen to death in his tent not far from our route. The small glacier looked steep and icy. We roped ourselves, improvising with my slings tied together. Santiago walked in the lead with one of my crampons on his right boot and a pair of ski poles for balance. I walked in the middle with the other crampon on my left boot. Rodrigo held my ice axe in the rear. I was skeptical about the safety of our arrangement. The soldiers' nonchalance offered little consolation—yet turning back now seemed worse than taking our chances crossing the glacier.

Using supreme powers of concentration to avoid a single misstep, we managed to make it safely to the other side without sliding down the glacier. We breathed a collective sigh of relief. But our relief didn't last long. A few yards further up the trail, we encountered a large, icy patch that was not yet melted by the morning sun.

As we carefully crossed the stretch of ice, I noticed that Rodrigo was only halfheartedly belaying us, with the point of my ice axe barely penetrating the ice. When I protested, he silenced me, saying that he knew what he was doing and had more experience in the mountains than I had.

Less than two minutes after our exchange of words, Santiago lost his footing and shot like a bolt of lightning down the steep slope, pulling Rodrigo and me behind him. My only thought was, "Oh God. We're all going to die."

Rodrigo managed to arrest our near-fatal fall by slamming the ice axe into the icy slope—but not until we had fallen several feet. The fall left us shaken but unhurt, with Rodrigo a little less arrogant. We lost a precious hour and precious energy in recovering our route. What a relief when we finally stepped onto dirt, rock, and gravel again, and could remove the slings that tied us together.

The brothers' pace slowed even more. They took big gasps of air between each step. Every 20 minutes or so, I stopped and waited for them to catch up.

While waiting for them, I had time to reflect on the austere, inhospitable grandeur surrounding me. My heart nearly burst with emotion, grateful that places like this still existed on our ravaged planet. I felt an irresistible urge to pray to the mountains, sun, sky, and rocks, and give thanks for the opportunity to experience the celestial world around me. I suppressed an urge to weep. I knew I had to contain myself to keep from depleting my carefully rationed store of energy. I whispered, "I love you, mountains. When I am with you, I feel the presence of the Holy Spirit." As I turned to continue walking, I felt a sense of grief that Mateo and I weren't able to share this magnificent grandeur together.

To the west, I could see the Pacific Ocean, a thin, blue line on the horizon. For a few miles in the same direction, I could see a big stretch of Chilean land below me.

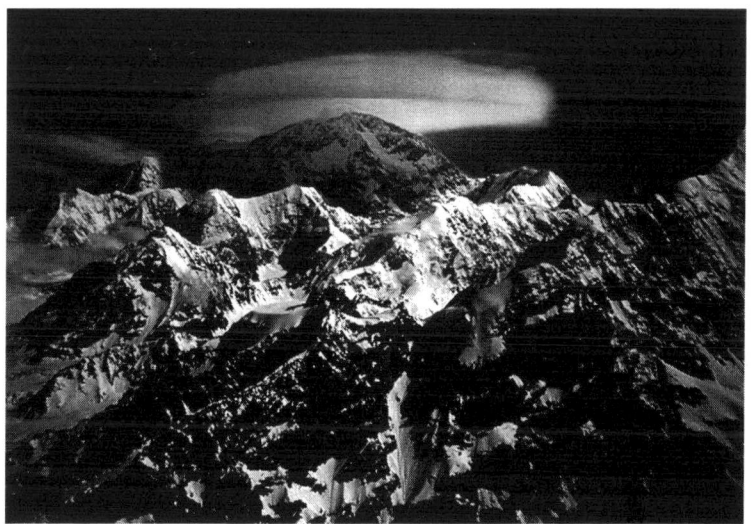

View of the surrounding mountains

Rows of jagged, saw-toothed mountains surrounded us. Not far to the south, an airplane had crashed in 1972. Sixteen members of the Uruguayan rugby team survived 70 days in sub-zero weather in the Andes, having to resort to cannibalism of their frozen friends to keep from starving to death. Being in the general vicinity gave me an even fuller appreciation of the survivors' courage. Their riveting story is recounted in the book *Alive*.

With the morning sun came perfect weather, with neither wind nor clouds. At eleven-thirty we arrived at the *canaleta*, or corridor, the most dreaded part of the climb. The steep, wide channel of rocks and boulders left us with no firm ground to place our feet. Dozens of rocks slipped downward *en masse* with each step. Progress was painfully slow, causing us high levels of frustration and further exhaustion. Because of the rarefied atmosphere, the summit looked deceptively close. What looked like it should take minutes in fact took hours of hard labor.

Most accidents on Aconcagua occur in the *canaleta*. Some people lose their minds and become hysterical, some fight each other, and some freeze to death. The thought crossed my mind, "What if the brothers turn on me? I'll be sure not to say anything they could take the wrong way."

Marcelo, the Ecuadorian climber, had hallucinated in the *canaleta*, imagining he saw shiny crosses. Rosa Maria, the Mexican climber from the beer company, screamed. Santiago had told me earlier in the climb about a rescue operation he had led to recover the body of a Japanese climber. They found the dead Japanese man seated outside his tent in his underwear, frozen, surely a victim of delirium.

The two brothers showed clear signs they were reaching the end of their strength. Their breathing turned into desperate panting for air. They took each step in slow motion and with the utmost care to conserve their strength. After every three steps, they rested, Rodrigo bending over my ice axe and Santiago leaning on his ski poles, muttering torrents of curse words between gasps of air. When I made a harmless comment, he told me to shut up, saying, "*Cállate, carajo.*"

Fortunately, my breathing remained under control. My body and mind still functioned well despite the strain, thanks to the multiple opportunities I'd had to acclimatize myself over the past weeks.

During my experiences climbing in Ecuador, I discovered that my body was capable of far more than I ever could have imagined. And the mind, I concluded, also plays a powerful role when it comes to endurance and survival. Now I had a chance to test that assumption. I had so thoroughly prepared myself psychologically to expect the worst on our climb that what I encountered on the mountain did not throw me off balance or terrify me.

As we neared the summit, I heard Santiago yelling something at me. I sat down on the only firm rock I could find and waited for the brothers to catch up. Although they were only a stone's throw away, it took them 20 minutes to get close enough so I could understand what they were yelling about. Their faces were swollen and ash-colored. Santiago yelled breathlessly, "Stop, *Gringa*. You need to listen to me. I'm boss of this expedition. Tomás isn't your boss anymore." When I asked him why he was so angry, he continued, "I'm going to get to the summit first, understand? You second."

Exhaustion had brought his competitive nature to a head. My mind flashed to the blood-chilling stories I'd heard about climbers becoming irritable and fighting each other, sometimes until death. "I don't care who gets to the summit first," I said with total sincerity.

This only made him angrier. "Don't fool me, *Gringa*. You want to get to the summit first to get the silver plaque the Mexicans left."

Rather than risk violence, I said nothing and stayed behind. I found their rhythm of resting every two feet much more exhausting than my slow but steady pace. But at this point, they had little alternative since they had so thoroughly burned themselves out from their fast pace when they started out in the morning, most likely trying to show off for me.

Just 100 feet below the summit, the brothers said they could go no further and I should go on by myself. I felt sorry that they would stop this close to their goal. I convinced them to get on their feet and give it one last try.

With my pushing, pulling, and constant encouragement, we arrived on the rocky summit at three-thirty that afternoon. We hugged each other briefly and then staggered around, too stunned to fully appreciate what we had done. Everything had a dream-like, ethereal quality, as though I was on some strange, mind-altering drug. Nothing seemed real anymore. I could feel my mind eluding me. I knew I must hasten to get us off the summit before we deteriorated beyond hope.

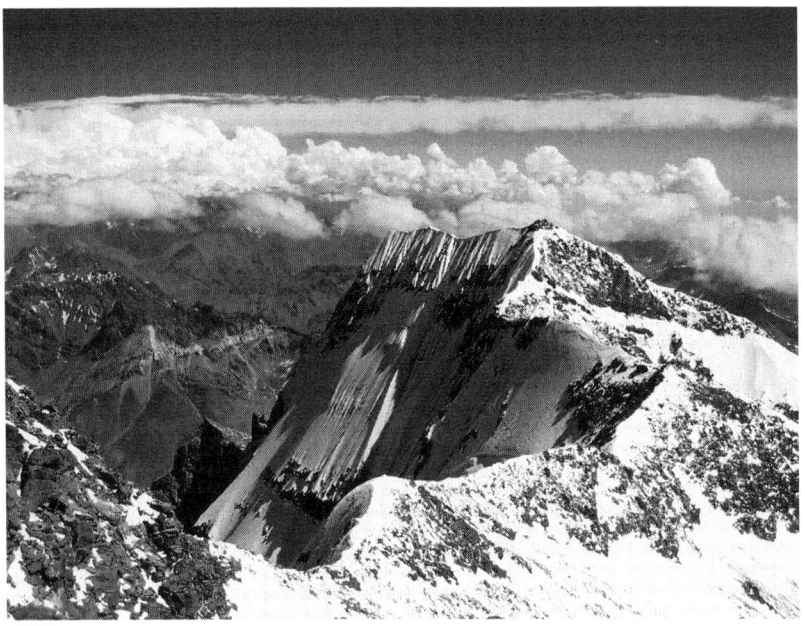

As I stood on the summit of Aconcagua, I stared in awe at the formidable South Wall just a few yards away.

Santiago found the silver plaque left by the Mexicans, which he had obsessed about on the climb, and put it in our backpack. Rodrigo took the banner of the beer company that had sponsored the Mexican expedition. I was left with a little silk flag of Mexico. We, in turn, left a banner, a bracelet, and two flags, one of Ecuador and one of Argentina. We put them in a plastic bag and left them in the little steel box containing the summit book. We signed the summit book on two pages, one of which we tore out to take to the army base as proof of our ascent, as was the custom. We placed the box under two large rocks.

My mind became increasingly foggy. It dimly occurred to me that I must take some pictures. The normally simple act of opening my pack, removing the camera, then adjusting the settings became a major undertaking. After regulating the aperture and shutter speed, I handed the camera to Santiago, who lay sprawled on the ground, and told him to just point the camera in my direction and press the button.

My next big project involved photographing all the cardinal points. Behind us loomed the dramatic South Wall, a massive sheet of rock that extended thousands of feet. My tired mind could barely comprehend the spectacular view.

We began our descent after spending a total of 15 minutes on the summit. My heart began pounding furiously in my chest. I developed a fierce headache.

The brothers had no strength left. They staggered and repeatedly lost their balance on the loose rocks. Progress was hopelessly slow. The afternoon wore on. Each time they fell, I prodded them to get up again. They insisted that I should let them "take a nap." They had lost their will.

I pleaded with them to keep going. We finally got to about 1,000 feet above Berlin when Santiago announced categorically that we had to bivouac. If we bivouacked, we would surely freeze to death since we had no bivouac gear with us—no tent, sleeping bag, or down pants in our pack.

When I begged them to keep walking, they told me to leave them alone. Night was not far away. I had to make a decision fast.

I left them lying on the ground and ran for help as fast as my trembling legs would permit. Just above the Berlin shelter, I ran into two of the former soldiers, Willy Noll and Luis. They had taken a short climb above Berlin to get acclimatized.

After several minutes trying to catch my breath, I managed to say breathlessly, "I need your help." My teeth chattered and my legs trembled uncontrollably. I had to lie down on the ground.

While trying to recover my speech, the two men took photographs of me lying on the ground. When I saw the prints weeks later in Buenos Aires, I understood why the men were so fascinated by my appearance. My entire body had become swollen like a beached whale. My skin looked grey and my eyes appeared wild behind slit, puffy eyelids.

After relating an abbreviated version of what happened, I urgently requested that they help Santiago and Rodrigo before they froze to death. The two men hastily climbed up to where they found the brothers lying on the ground in a stupor. With difficulty, they helped Santiago and Rodrigo stagger down to the Berlin shelter. They arrived at the shelter at ten o'clock that night, in the dark without their headlamps.

The brothers looked like wild men, utterly exhausted, incoherent, and dehydrated. That evening Willy Noll gave each of us a total of three liters of liquid to alleviate our severe dehydration. Santiago and Rodrigo, unable to speak, just drank their liquid while staring off into space. Willy and Luis had to put them into their sleeping bags as though they were helpless children. Several times in the night, we had to nudge them awake from nightmares. We could hear them kicking in their sleeping bags and gasping for breath, as though reliving some of the trauma of the day before.

As I unpacked my backpack, I noticed that we had not eaten a single morsel of food all day, except for a handful of honey drops.

The next morning, we ate our first meal in 36 hours. Liquids were the only substance our bodies craved. Digesting food just added to our bodies' demand for oxygen, which was already seriously insufficient at this altitude.

The next day, Santiago and Rodrigo left Berlin and headed for base camp at Plaza de Mulas to more fully recuperate. Willy Noll and Luis headed up the mountain to the summit. I stayed alone in Berlin in case someone needed help in an emergency.

At two-thirty that afternoon, I heard shouts. After a few minutes I could see Raúl staggering toward Berlin, accompanied by Alberto. They told me they had gotten as far as Independencia when Raúl became sick from *puna* and could go no further. I agreed to accompany them down the mountain. At five-thirty we left the shelter for Plaza Vieja. They needed constant encouragement to keep up their pace. Darkness fell. We had no headlamps with us. Fortunately the route was very familiar to me.

We arrived at Plaza Vieja a little after ten o'clock and found Tomás asleep, along with climbers from another expedition out of Córdoba, Argentina. Our arrival woke the climbers. We all conversed about the day's events until we could no longer stay awake.

Tomás, Alberto, and I decided to sleep outside under the stars. When they thought I was asleep, they began to talk softly with each other. Tomás cried because his son hadn't made it to the top. He said he felt embarrassed because his expedition had received so much publicity and no one had made the summit from his group. He threatened to go back up the mountain to try again. His son, understandably concerned, tried to reason with him, saying that he was too old to keep climbing this mountain. Tomás replied that he wouldn't mind leaving his body on the mountain.

Poor Alberto, in his frustration, "woke" me up to help in persuading his father to go home. I had no more success than Alberto. Finally I offered to accompany Tomás back up the mountain, but he would hear nothing of it, preferring to go alone.

With sad hearts, Raúl, Alberto, and I said goodbye to Tomás the next morning. We arrived at Plaza de Mulas and found the base camp filled with climbers, including two expeditions from Mendoza, one American expedition (all sick with *puna*), and one from Spain.

Some of the climbers stood up when I walked through the door, cheered, and gave me congratulatory hugs. They had heard of *la mujer Americana* from other climbers. News had also spread to soldiers at the army base at Puente de Inca.

The climbers celebrated me as *Cabra Montés* (Mountain Goat) and treated me to a delicious meal prepared by the Spaniards' private cook. Ravenous and gaunt, I ate with gusto and enthusiastically accepted seconds and thirds, which pleased the cook. Later, at base camp, I got on the doctor's scale and discovered that I had lost around 15 pounds since the physical exam I had with my Ecuadorian *compañeros*.

Raúl, Alberto, and I followed the river out of the valley two days later. The young men walked very slowly, still exhausted from being on the mountain so long. When we reached Lake Horcones, three families came out to meet me with big hugs and smiles. They were Argentine tourists who had heard that an American woman had made it to the top. They brought me a bottle of wine and a basket of food and then photographed me.

I felt awkward at having such a fuss made over me. At the army base the officers treated me like a celebrity, probably because it was so unusual in South America at that time for women to climb in the mountains, the once-exclusive domain of men. Everyone I ran into wanted to shake my hand. People gave me presents: a ring, a bracelet, and a hand-painted ashtray. Why an ashtray? Even Argentinian climbers loved their cigarettes. The major gave me free room and board. One of the soldiers washed my clothes and polished my boots.

The major invited me to have dinner with him and his wife. He proposed a toast to me and announced that I was the first American woman with proof of reaching the summit. He said an American woman had climbed Aconcagua solo in 1974. She claimed to have reached the summit. The major said she had no evidence to prove her claim—no photos, no souvenir taken from the summit, no notation in the summit book.

The next afternoon a local family walked with me to the cemetery where the bodies of the climbers who didn't make it are buried. I got chills standing in the cemetery and gave thanks to God that I had come out alive.

I read the newspaper article about our climb. I noted that Santiago and Rodrigo had not reported any of the details—simply that they had reached the summit. Perhaps they were too embarrassed to say what really happened. In another paper, there was no mention that I was with them at all.

In Santiago, Chile, I shipped my equipment back to the States and began my travels around the South American continent. Thoughts of Tomás weighed heavily on my mind. Then my worst fears came true when I read in the newspaper that he had been reported dead. The thought was unbearable to me. After several days I telephoned his family to give my condolences and discovered, to my huge relief, that the news report had been a false alarm. Tomás had been stranded in a snowstorm near Berlin for six days. He lost 40 pounds but came out alive. His reputation as a diehard was well earned.

During my travels, I visited Tomás and the rest of our group, along with the priests and some of the other people who befriended me on the mountain, including Rosa Maria in Mexico, just before I crossed over into the States.

Chapter 29

ON THE ROAD

In Santiago, right before I embarked on my long journey homeward, I treated myself to a delicious lunch in an upscale restaurant. While I was eating, a family seated next to my table spontaneously engaged me in conversation. When I told them I had recently climbed Aconcagua and intended to travel around South America, the father suggested that I ride with his family to Patagonia, where he owned a ranch on several hundred acres of untamed land. He said I would see some of the most spectacular mountain scenery in the world, including glacial fjords and rugged, unclimbed peaks.

Patagonia, a sparsely populated region at that time, encompasses the southernmost tip of South America. The Andes mountain range divides the Argentine side from the Chilean side.

I stayed with the Chilean family for a few days, thoroughly enjoying their warm hospitality. I rode horseback with the boys, participated in their daily chores, and helped the mother prepare hearty meals—all the while marveling at the pristine countryside.

One of the sons offered to drive me to the Argentine side of Patagonia to a province called "Tierra del Fuego," the Land of Fire, named after the signaling fires used by the original inhabitants of the area. We spent the day together exploring the stunning region. At the end of the day, the young man dropped me off at a youth hostel in a village called Ushuaia, located on the southernmost tip of South America.

In the youth hostel, I met a friendly American backpacker who had taken a year off to travel before going to medical school. We spent a couple days roaming around together in Tierra del Fuego, marveling at the wild beauty of nature, and then we went our separate ways, reconnecting briefly years later when he was a practicing medical doctor.

While in Ushuaia, I hiked in the rugged and stunningly beautiful countryside surrounding the village. The magnificence of the mountains and the vastness of the ocean filled me with awe and reverence.

I walked to the southernmost tip and looked out over the Beagle Channel toward Antarctica. I vowed that someday I would find a way to go there.

Although the water was freezing, I took off my clothes down to my skimpy underwear and jumped into the Beagle Channel. I swam for a few icy minutes, just for the thrill of it. I dried myself off as best I could with an extra T-shirt in my backpack, got dressed, and then walked over to where the ships came into port.

As I stood watching, I saw a ship arrive and the passengers disembark down the plank. When the captain walked past me, I said, on impulse, "Excuse me, Sir. Can you please tell me if it would be possible for me to get a job in Antarctica?" He answered, "Certainly. We'd be glad to have you."

With excitement in my voice, I asked what kinds of jobs would be available for me. He said that for any job I took, I would have to sign a contract, agreeing to work for a minimum of a full year. With that news, my interest vanished. I needed to eventually get home and see my family.

I could have stayed in Tierra del Fuego for months of exploration, but I wanted to see the rest of the continent. One of the backpackers I met at the youth hostel urged me to take a bus to an alpine town called Bariloche, located in the northern part of Patagonia and considered one of the most scenic places in all of Argentina. He said that Bariloche resembled an alpine village in Switzerland or Germany, with dozens of mountain lakes and towering snow-covered peaks nearby.

I took a bus to Bariloche and stayed in an inexpensive hostel designated for mountain climbers. The following morning I joined a small group of German hikers and spent the day high in the Andes, walking in the snowfields.

On the second day of my stay, I wandered around the town, noting how similar the architecture was to that found in Europe. I knew that many Europeans had immigrated to Argentina after World War II—including a significant number of former Nazis.

In the afternoon I decided to go to an expensive hotel with a fabulous view of the mountains and treat myself to a cup of tea, a luxury I could barely afford.

I sat by myself at a table on the balcony, enchanted by the view of a crystalline blue lake and jagged mountains in the distance. At the next table, middle-aged German men spoke loudly among themselves. One of them looked over at me and said, in a heavy accent, "Hello, Miss. How are you?" I answered him back in my schoolgirl German. A conversation ensued. They asked me where I learned to speak German. When I told them I spent my high school years in Germany and that my mother was Swiss, they became very friendly and invited me to join their table.

When I asked them what they did in World War II, the men spoke freely about being Nazis and working for the SS. I could not detect even a trace of shame, remorse, or secrecy. One of the German men said, "Did you know that after the war the American government invited quite a few Nazis with specific skills to immigrate to the United States to help Americans fight communism, head corporations, and work with American scientists on various projects?" They mentioned a rocket scientist, Werner von Braun. My father had been one of his associates and spoke very highly of him. I'm sure my father had no idea that Von Braun had worked for the Nazi Party.

After several minutes of awkward conversation, I realized it was time to excuse myself. I wished them well and departed.

After spending a few days in Buenos Aires, I headed to Brazil. On the way, I stopped to marvel at the breathtaking falls of Iguazú, the largest waterfall in the world, twice as tall as Niagara Falls and three times as wide, on the border between Argentina and Brazil.

While camping near the falls, I met Louisa, an attractive, longhaired British woman about my age. She had hitchhiked around the continent by herself. To keep safe, she only accepted rides from families. She asked if I would like to hitchhike with her to Rio de Janeiro for Carnival, a huge festival held every year before Lent, the equivalent of Mardi Gras in New Orleans. I agreed to go with her.

We waited only about ten minutes by the side of the road when a family stopped and picked us up. When we told them we were headed to Rio, they said they were going there as well to celebrate Carnival. After a friendly conversation among us, the family said that they had some friends who could put Louisa and me up for a few nights and even feed us while we visited Rio de Janeiro.

Nothing had prepared me for what I witnessed in Rio. The streets overflowed with colorful floats, revelers in outrageous costumes, and continuous dance contests sponsored by various samba schools. The air vibrated with sensuous samba music that created an irresistible urge to dance with abandon.

Our hosts said that everyone participates in this yearly extravaganza, even the desperately poor people in the *favelas*—the slums on hills throughout the city. Even though they barely have enough money to survive, each year they saved up what they could to buy the fabric for creating their own elaborate costumes. The costumes and music were a mix of colonial Europe, Indigenous, and Afro-Brazilian. Every shade of skin color, from porcelain white to deep black, could be seen on the streets.

After two days of intense participation in Carnival, Louisa and I were ready for a break. We headed to the beach. From my towel, I watched the people walking up and down the beach. I observed a large range of body types, from slender to corpulent. The way the women held themselves as they walked along the beach intrigued me. Even middle-aged and older women, with rolls of adipose tissue hanging over their skimpy bikinis, looked beautiful to me. They walked as though they were listening to some internal source of dance music, with heads held high, hips swinging, giving the impression of being proud and happy to be alive. I concluded that simple happiness and joy adds more to one's beauty than any kind of makeup or cosmetic procedure.

Louisa stayed on in Rio de Janeiro after I left to slowly traverse the continent from east to west on my way back to Quito, Ecuador, where I hoped to reconnect with Mateo before heading home to the States. Over the next three months, I spent time exploring the luscious and exuberant rainforest in Brazil and the mountainous villages and ruins in Bolivia and Peru.

When I finally reached the Ecuadorian border, I caught a direct bus to Quito. During the long bus ride, I could hardly contain my excitement thinking about seeing Mateo again.

The bus depot in Quito was located not too far from the company that had published my bilingual storybook. When I dropped by, the publisher gave me a big smile as he handed me a copy of the softback book with the student's simple black-and-white drawing on the front. What a gratifying feeling to see the published version of the bilingual book project! The publisher shook my hand vigorously and thanked me for my dedication in helping *los Indios*.

I stuffed the book into my backpack and headed to the Peace Corps office to pick up my last paycheck and make a few phone calls to friends and family. I eagerly anticipated talking to Mateo and spending precious time with him—maybe two or three weeks—before I continued my travels. I fantasized about him meeting up with me in the States someday.

I dialed Mateo's number. His sister answered the phone.

"*Aló. Con quien hablo?*" Hello, to whom am I speaking? She spoke without any emotion in her voice.

"Hello. This is Erica Elliott. May I please speak with your brother, Mateo?"

The sister's response left me speechless.

With fire in her voice, she said, "You may not speak to Mateo. In fact, I don't want you to ever call here again. Do you understand?"

I remained too stunned to speak.

She continued, "Mateo never saw the letters you wrote to him. I tore them up."

"Why did you do that?"

"Why? Don't you have any idea why? Mateo has fallen in love with you. If he leaves us to be with you in America, we will have no way to survive. He is our hope. We depend on him to take us out of poverty."

She began to cry. Through her sobs, she said, "Please leave us alone. Do not call or write."

Her tears softened my state of shock. In a choked-up voice I said to her, "I'm so sorry I've been the cause of such distress in your family. I will go now. Goodbye."

I sat on the couch in the Peace Corps office in a daze, trying to digest the contents of the phone call. The idea of never having any contact with Mateo again seemed unbearable and left me with a feeling of emptiness. I couldn't hold back the tears.

The Peace Corps nurse noticed my state of grief as she walked past and asked what was wrong. After I explained briefly what happened, she said she had something that would cheer me up. She went into her office and returned with a newspaper article she had saved for me. The featured article on the front page of the Sunday supplement of *El Comercio* was a story about our Ecuadorian climb of Aconcagua, including photos. I carefully folded the newspaper and slid it into a side pocket of my backpack. I gave hugs to the volunteers in the office and headed back to the bus station.

On the bus, I met a delightful young Danish couple who had taken a year off to travel the world. We became instant friends, as though we had known each other our whole lives. I shared with them briefly about my time in the Peace Corps and my current heartache over Mateo. They convinced me to go with them to an island off the coast of Colombia, called San Andrés.

Both the Caribbean island and the Danish couple were so enchanting that I ended up staying for two weeks. We spent our days walking along the beach with pink-colored sand, snorkeling in pristine water, marveling at the coral reefs and the schools of colorful fish, listening to reggae and calypso music, and dancing to the point of near collapse. We rented bicycles and pedaled the entire perimeter of the island. The Danes knew how to have fun.

After forming a strong bond, we decided to stay together during our month-long journey through Central America. We parted ways in Mexico. The Danish couple headed back to Europe, and I headed to my parents' home in New Hampshire. We remained friends for many years.

I caught a Greyhound bus at the US border and headed north and eastward. I made many short stops along the way to visit siblings and old friends from my past. My trip across the States was fast, with the goal of getting home as soon as possible.

I did not foresee the disorienting culture shock that I would face upon my return home.

Chapter 30

BACK HOME

I FINALLY ARRIVED AT MY PARENTS' HOME in New Hampshire after nearly seven months of travel since leaving the Peace Corps. My parents were excited to see me—relieved that I had returned safe and sound.

My mother had an upsetting scare when she received a phone call from the American Embassy in Quito, Ecuador, around the time I was climbing Aconcagua. The official on the other end of the phone insisted on speaking to my father and, for some unknown reason, would not reveal to my mother the nature of the call. While my mother waited for my father to return from the college where he worked, she cried, assuming that the Embassy was going to tell them their daughter had died on Aconcagua. The Embassy simply wanted to know my whereabouts after I left the Peace Corps.

My mother expressed her love for me by cooking delicious meals and arranging a series of parties with various groups of my parents' friends in the community, most of whom I didn't know.

After the excitement of returning home wore off, I felt out of sorts, verging on depression. I had an overwhelming sense of isolation and disconnection, as though I was a stranger in a foreign country. The rampant materialism and tremendous waste in the United States added to my sense of malaise.

Behind those feelings of disconnection and loneliness was a pervasive sense of grief that I might never again see Mateo.

I called up a good friend from my Peace Corps group. She reported having similar difficulties with re-entry. We both felt disoriented, with feelings of emptiness. We found ourselves tearful for no apparent reason. We decided that we had "reverse culture shock." We also admitted that we might be experiencing the normal letdown that comes after living a meaningful life of service, where every minute held something new and exciting.

Usually culture shock comes from being assigned to a country that bears little resemblance to one's own country. We were warned during our orientation that we might experience culture shock and that it would eventually pass. We were not warned about the shock that can happen upon returning home to one's country of origin.

> *What do I do with my life? Where do I go from here?*
> *Where do I belong? I feel lost.*

One morning I got up early, after a restless night of sleep, and tiptoed downstairs, trying not to wake my parents. I thought that if I did an hour of yoga, it would help lift my spirits. After about ten minutes, I gave up the yoga, lay prone on the thick Persian rug in the living room, and began to cry with my face supported on my folded arms.

Within minutes, my father's voice startled me. He stood in the doorway in his pajamas and asked why I was crying. Overcome with embarrassment, I mumbled that I'd had a bad night. He persisted, "What's wrong, Rickie?" I confessed to him that I felt completely lost and that my life seemed meaningless, without any purpose. I also confessed that I missed Mateo terribly, but I couldn't call him because his family didn't want me to have any contact with him, afraid that they would lose him.

My father's response stunned me. Focusing on my perceived lack of purpose, he said, "Rickie, I suggest you put your energy into becoming a medical doctor. I've noticed that you have a natural propensity for helping people feel better. You'd be an excellent doctor. Don't forget that your Uncle Ernst and your grandfather were both Swiss doctors. Medicine is in your blood."

I answered emphatically, "Are you joking, Daddy? I'm not nearly as smart as Uncle Ernst. He's a genius. I'm definitely not a genius. I could never be a doctor like him. Maybe I'll go to massage school and learn how to help people feel better that way."

"You think about what I said, okay?" he said with gravitas in his voice. He left the living room and went into the kitchen to brew some coffee. I thought about what he said for about two minutes and then dismissed the idea as unrealistic.

During those miserable days of existential anguish, I received a letter from the Admissions office at Antioch College offering me a temporary job.

The college had hired a man named Roy Smith to run their leadership program in outdoor education. The college asked him to arrange an orientation program in the wilderness for incoming freshmen. Having read about my expeditions in South America in the Antioch alumni magazine, Roy wanted to hire me to lead a group of freshmen students on a weeklong wilderness trip in the Smoky Mountains as part of their orientation before they began classes.

I readily accepted the offer, thinking that maybe the experience would lead me in the general direction of my life's purpose— although I still didn't have any idea what that purpose was. I only knew some of the characteristics that my purpose needed to include, like sharing information and knowledge that would empower people and make a meaningful difference in their lives.

The weeklong wilderness trip in the Great Smoky Mountains National Park grounded me and gave me a temporary sense of purpose. I noted how rewarding it was to share my love of the wilderness with the students and watch the beneficial effects it had on them. My favorite part was sitting around the campfire at the end of the day and sharing stories about our lives. By the end of the trip, the students had formed a tight bond with each other.

Roy phoned me at my parents' home to discuss the wilderness orientation experience. He praised me for how I handled the leadership role with the freshmen and told me it was a big success, according to the feedback the students had given. He said I had a natural talent for teaching "experiential education," and he strongly encouraged me to pursue this field.

I assumed that what Roy meant by experiential education was learning important lessons about life through one's direct experiences, especially in the great outdoors.

He suggested I get in touch with a friend and colleague of his in Boulder, Colorado, named Joe Nold, a legendary figure in the field of experiential education. Among Joe's many accomplishments was his role as founding director of Colorado Outward Bound School, or COBS.

Joe wanted to bring the principles taught in Outward Bound to higher education. He created a master's degree program in experiential education at the University of Colorado (CU) in Boulder. Roy said I would get accepted with no problem because I was the kind of candidate that Joe was looking for.

While hiking in the Great Smoky Mountains, I had fantasized about starting a wilderness school for teens and young adults who were having difficulties at home and in school. I realized that to fulfill this dream, I would need a graduate degree in outdoor education.

I wrote Joe a letter asking to join the master's program and gave my reasons why. I included an abbreviated description of my background. As soon as Joe received the letter, he called me on the phone and welcomed me into his program.

I could hardly believe how fast my future was unfolding, with so little effort on my part. Joe asked me to be in Boulder by the following week. I agreed and made arrangements to drive across the country.

Through my studies with Joe Nold, I met Jeff Lowe, a renowned alpine climber and co-owner, with his brothers, of Lowe Outdoor Gear. Jeff gave me private lessons in ice climbing. He lent me the special gear I needed to ascend vertical ice walls formed by frozen waterfalls.

Jeff introduced me to his world of climbing friends, one of whom was a man named Jerry who had organized an expedition to climb Mt. Everest the following year. Jerry had read an article I wrote about my climb of Aconcagua, published in the climbing magazine *Mountain Gazette*. He got in touch and invited me to join his expedition, which meant that I would have to commit to an intense training program to get into shape. Jerry also convinced me to sign up for a weeklong avalanche search-and-rescue training course in the Grand Tetons, near Jackson Hole, Wyoming.

The training program that Jerry had designed required a commitment of about three hours a day. The routines included runs up the side of nearby mountains at the crack of dawn. While training, I felt some serious doubts about participating in his expedition. Jerry's approach seemed grim, overly serious, and ultra-competitive. I missed the laughter, the joy, and the sense of camaraderie I had with my climbing partners in Ecuador.

During one of the training sessions, I twisted my ankle and ripped two of the ligaments that hold the joint in place, requiring me to use crutches and a brace for a month. I felt my body was trying to tell me something. I quit the training and told Jerry I wanted to put my focus elsewhere.

Less than a year later, I heard from Jeff Lowe that three of the people on Jerry's Everest expedition had died in an avalanche. I thanked my body for my sprained ankle.

After I'd completed one semester in the experiential education master's program, Joe Nold encouraged me to sign up as a student on an upcoming OB course in Canyonlands, Utah. He wanted me to witness how the course exemplified the concepts of experiential education in action. He thought that I would love the experience and would consider being an instructor for Outward Bound in the summers.

From Outward Bound's promotional literature, I learned that the organization's roots went back to the early 1940s when an influential educator and philosopher, Kurt Hahn, developed a survival training program for British sailors, based on the philosophy that confronting challenges had the potential to produce the best character traits in the men.

In 1962, a man named Josh Miner adopted Hahn's philosophy and founded Outward Bound USA in Marble, Colorado, where COBS still operates to this day.

As Joe Nold predicted, I did indeed become hooked after my first Outward Bound experience and agreed to spend my summers instructing for COBS. I accepted the job with the hope that I could make a difference in the students' lives by helping them get a glimpse of their full potential. Based on my own experience, I knew that the mountains and the wilderness could be the perfect classroom for significant inner growth and transformation.

Chapter 31

OUTWARD BOUND

ON THE EDGE OF A BIG MEADOW, with the Sangre de Cristo Mountains looming in the background, I waited for the students to arrive. A herd of antelope grazed peacefully in the distance. Piles of backpacks and other mountaineering gear lay on the ground around me. The bus that Outward Bound had rented approached in the distance. When the bus came to a stop, nine Outward Bound students emerged, carrying their suitcases. Most of the students looked eager in anticipation. A few looked apprehensive.

I vividly remember that first course as an instructor in June of 1977. The course took place in southern Colorado in the Sangre de Cristo Mountains, a section of the 3,000-mile Rocky Mountain range that extends all the way to northern New Mexico.

I welcomed the students to the 23-day Outward Bound expedition. After we learned each other's names, we sat on the ground in a circle to hear my orientation talk:

"This course might be the most difficult experience you have ever had in your life. You will be challenged on all levels—physically, mentally, and emotionally. The course will not be easy, but it will be worth it. At the end of the 23 days, you might feel like you've become a different person. In fact, your parents might wonder what happened to you!" The students laughed in unison—a nervous kind of laughter.

As part of the orientation, I asked the students to participate in an experiment in which none of us would reveal anything about ourselves for the first three days, other than our first names. I wanted all of the students to start on a level playing field, without any preconceived ideas about each other.

I came up with this idea after reviewing their bios in advance and discovering that I had an unusual array of students. The oldest student, Jerome, was a 60-year-old recently retired MIT professor who had no prior wilderness experience and had never carried a backpack. He wanted to challenge himself at this major crossroad and get some perspective on where to go with his post-retirement life.

One of the two youngest students, Jackson, was a 16-year-old member of an inner-city gang who frequently got into trouble with the law. A progressive judge in the juvenile justice system astutely recognized Jackson's untapped potential and gave him the option of attending an Outward Bound course instead of serving time in a juvenile detention center.

That same judge encouraged another 16-year-old boy on the list, named Luc, to take an Outward Bound course. Luc was raised in France until he was eight, when his family moved to the United States. Luc was extremely intelligent and creative, with an overactive imagination. After watching American movies about bank robberies, he decided to play a prank on his local bank. He rode his bicycle to the drive-up window, pulled out his plastic squirt gun, and told the cashier to give him the money. Instead of getting a good laugh, he got arrested by the police.

After our get-acquainted circle, I described what a typical day might look like. It meant getting up at dawn, making breakfast, packing up camp and leaving it as pristine as when we arrived, mapping the route, and then heading out. The hiking might be all day, broken up with short breaks to rest, snack, and enjoy the spectacular views.

Rest stops also served as teaching opportunities, especially regarding the area's history, geology, flora, and fauna.

I went on to say that our hiking might be on trails, but more often it would be "off trail," where we would learn to navigate through forests, rushing rivers, steep and rocky terrain, snow and ice, and the inevitable stormy mountain weather. Hiking off trail also gave us the opportunity to have a true wilderness experience, without running into hikers and climbers.

I introduced the students to their gear, which lay in piles on the grass, including backpacks, sleeping bags, pads, tarps, tents, helmets for rock climbing, ice axes, two climbing ropes, fresh and freeze-dried food, three portable gas cook stoves, pots and pans and other cooking utensils, down parkas, rain gear, flashlights, maps, and compasses.

I asked them to go through their suitcases and take out only what was absolutely essential on the expedition, besides their warm clothes, footgear, and toiletries. I could barely suppress a laugh when Cindy, one of the four young women on the course, asked if she could bring her portable hair dryer and her makeup kit. Another student, Allison, wanted to take clothing that was more appropriate for going on a date.

Jackson came up to me as I was distributing the gear and said, "Are you really our leader? I thought we were gonna get a man."

"Are you disappointed that your instructor is a woman?"

"Shit yeah! I don't wanna do some wimpy course with a lady."

"You don't need to worry about that, Jackson," I replied.

By the time they packed their gear in their backpacks and stacked their suitcases in the bus, it was time for a light lunch that Outward

Bound staff had provided and sent on the bus with the students. I passed out the sandwiches and fresh fruit to the group and asked them to fill their water bottles from a ten-gallon container on the bus.

After lunch I gave the students a briefing about the five-mile hike toward the foothills of the mountains. I described the meadow where we would set up camp near a mountain stream.

The students hoisted the 50-pound packs onto their backs. Some of them needed assistance. I heard a lot of moaning and groaning as they began hiking.

After an hour, Jackson breathlessly asked, "We almost at the meadow?" I answered, "We've only walked about one mile at the most." As he wiped the sweat off his forehead with his bandana, he grumbled, "Maybe I should have let the judge put me in jail instead of choosing this shit. Man, this is fucked."

After the groaning and panting subsided and they learned to set a pace they could sustain, the students began chattering among themselves about their favorite TV shows and movies they had seen. Although they stuck to my request not to discuss anything that would reveal their identities, I realized that the chattering was keeping them from noticing their surroundings.

As soon as we took a brief rest stop, I requested that they only talk about the present moment for the next three days. They didn't understand what I meant. I asked them to focus on what they were feeling, seeing, hearing, touching, and smelling. The ensuing silence felt refreshing—until it was punctured by complaints of fatigue, aches, and pains.

Just before sunset, the students staggered into the meadow. They took off their packs and lay sprawled out on the ground. Eventually they got up and started figuring out how to set up their tents.

I chose Jackson to share the tent with the professor. I sensed that they might learn a lot from each other. I assigned the three other men a tent designed to accommodate more people. The four women paired up in the remaining two-person tents. I set up my own one-person tent out of sight, behind a clump of bushes, about 100 feet away from the group.

While the students put up their tents and made their sleeping arrangements, I set up a makeshift kitchen and started assembling the dinner with the packets of freeze-dried meat and veggies, dried herbs and spices, rice, and a thick tahini sauce. We had freeze-dried strawberry shortcake for dessert. The students ate like they were starving. Out in the wilderness, even freeze-dried food tastes delicious.

After dinner the students refilled their water bottles with filtered stream water. I asked them to divvy up the camping food, including their own personal stash, and put the items in food bags. We used the climbing ropes to suspend the bags high off the ground in order to avoid attracting bears to our campsite.

We ended the day sitting on the ground around the campfire, taking turns talking about our thoughts and feelings. Mandy, Cindy, and Allison expressed concern that they would not be able to complete the 23-day course. Cindy said, "If I had known that the course was this hard, there's no way in Hell I would have agreed to participate."

Cindy, age 22, came at her parents' urging. She could not hold down a job more than a few months, was preoccupied with clothes, makeup, dating, and watching TV shows. Her parents wrote that she was a "lost soul" looking for some direction in life.

Mandy was a 19-year-old college dropout with an eating disorder, and about 30 pounds overweight. She had no experience in the wilderness and appeared frightened about what lay ahead on the course.

Allison, age 24, struggled with alcoholism. She came from an extremely wealthy family that bought her whatever she wanted. She still lived with her parents and never had to work. Her counselor recommended that she sign up for an OB course to help her find meaning and purpose in her life.

The three young women concluded that the course was too difficult for them. I sensed that others in the group had the same unexpressed concerns. I reassured them. "It's too early to make conclusions. You might be surprised to find out what you're capable of doing." I told the young women how proud I was of them making it this far. On that positive note, we all headed to our tents and crawled into our sleeping bags.

The next morning, the air was brisk as the sun appeared on the horizon. The roaring mountain stream next to the campsite had a natural pool about five feet deep and 12 feet wide. I woke up the students and let them know that jumping into the water was an invigorating way to start the day. Bathing suits were optional. Four of the students, three men and one woman, emerged from their tents in their underwear and jumped into the icy water with loud yelps.

When all the students gathered around the kitchen area, I told them, "Each day a different student will be the designated leader, helping the group get organized for breakfast, dish washing, breaking down camp, and cleaning up our campsite. During the day of hiking, that same person will lead the group up the mountain, relying on the topographical map and compass when there are no trail markers and when we are off trail." The students appeared to be confused about what I said.

"Jackson, you're going to be our first student leader," I announced.

"No way!" he protested.

I assured him that I would guide him, starting with making breakfast. Once Jackson learned that he could ask for assistance, he seemed less stressed. He and Jerome, his tent mate, worked on making breakfast and urging their fellow students to take down their tents and break camp while they waited for breakfast to be ready. Breakfast consisted of oatmeal and granola, topped with freeze-dried blueberries and reconstituted powdered milk. Jackson served each student a cup of coffee or herbal tea. I made a mental note of how much he seemed to enjoy being in charge.

After breakfast, Jackson, in his role as leader, made sure that the dishes got washed in boiled water from the stream, everyone's water bottles got filled, and the gear was packed up and ready to go. I gave a little class on how to use a map and compass for navigation. Since Jackson was the leader for the day, he would navigate us over unmarked terrain to our next campsite, a day's hike away, near the base of the 14,000-foot mountain that loomed over us.

During the hike, I observed the interpersonal dynamics of the group. I saw the students helping each other cross the slippery mountain streams and navigate rocky terrain. When we stopped for lunch, I heard Jackson offer to carry some of the contents of Jerome's pack when he saw Jerome staggering from exhaustion. Jackson became Jerome's lifeline, offering a hand whenever necessary. Jerome, on the other hand, became a wise and caring father figure for Jackson.

Cindy and Allison had bonded as well—in their dislike of being in the wilderness. They announced that they planned on turning around and finding a way to get back home. They listed all the things they hated about the trip, like wearing dirty clothes, having unwashed hair, digging makeshift latrines, having to sometimes use the leaves of certain plants as toilet paper in the name of low-impact camping, sleeping on the ground, hauling around a heavy backpack, hearing scary noises at night, fearing being attacked by bears and mountain lions, and missing their comfortable beds and their favorite foods. To my amazement, the rest of the group gave them earnest words of encouragement, revealing a surprising level of empathy and compassion. They eventually convinced the girls to hang in there. The group began to show the first signs of working as a team.

In the late afternoon we came to our campsite on the edge of an alpine lake. We arrived early enough to swim in the frigid water. The men took off all their clothes and dove headlong into the water. The four women left on their underwear and entered the water more cautiously. I heard lots of yelps, some of which sounded like expressions of sheer joy.

The scenery encircling our campsite struck us with its austere and majestic beauty. The students had become more aware of their surroundings and no longer needed constant reminding to return their attention to the here and now.

At every opportunity, I talked about the local geology and history of the region, as well as pointing out the names of the trees, shrubs, and the many colorful spring wildflowers. Vibrant swaths of reds and oranges created by the blooms of Indian paintbrush, and the blues and purples of the delicate columbines, bedazzled the students. Getting this kind of detailed orientation appeared to help the students feel more at home in the wilderness.

On the third day, I designated Patricia as leader of the day. Patricia, age 22, was a high achiever, top student, and a recent graduate from a well-known college. Without any outside prompting, she signed up for the OB course in order to challenge herself. A keen observer, she eagerly assumed her role as leader without needing much supervision. She was the perfect tent mate for Mandy.

The students spent most of the day learning how to rock climb on a wall of small cliffs, approximately 60 feet high. I gave a demonstration on how to tie specific kinds of knots, put on a climbing harness, use the carabiners and slings, and how to spot handholds and footholds. After I taught the students the rock climbing lingo, we donned our helmets and practiced what we had learned on the flat land until everyone felt comfortable to start climbing the rock wall—that is, everyone except Mandy. She had confessed to me at the beginning of the course that she had a deathly fear of heights. Patricia took Mandy aside and encouraged her to at least give rock climbing a try.

Mandy reluctantly agreed to give it a try on the condition that I would be the person belaying her from the top of the cliff. Jackson, without being asked, checked everyone's climbing gear before they started the climb. I hiked up to the top of the cliff, established an anchor for myself by tying one end of the rope around a nearby ponderosa pine tree, and then I threw down the rest of the 150-foot rope. Jackson carefully scrutinized Mandy's harness, carabiner, and knots to make sure she was securely tied into the rope.

At Mandy's request, Jackson held onto her body as she took her first tentative moves on the wall of the cliff. When she got six feet off the ground, Jackson could no longer maintain contact. Mandy let out a little scream. Every single student cheered her on, saying repeatedly, "You can do it. Hang in there, girl. Don't give up." She inched her way up about three more feet and then her legs began to tremble uncontrollably and she started hyperventilating. She yelled up at me, "I can't do this. Let me down." She rappelled to the ground and, through tears, she said, "Sorry guys, I let you down." After Jackson untied her, the group gathered around her and told her she did a good job and at least gave rock climbing a try. She got several heartfelt hugs from both the men and the women.

Cindy went next, followed by Allison. Each of them needed constant coaching and encouragement. With great effort and lots of advice from the students on the ground, they managed to reach the top. They were both shocked that they had been able to get all the way up—in spite of their fears and limiting beliefs about themselves. One after the other, they rappelled back down the little cliff. I could hear them screaming with delight. Once on the ground, I heard one of them yell up to me, "We did it!!!"

We went back to our campsite in a state of exhilaration, ate lunch, wrote in our journals, and then returned to spend the rest of the day doing more rock climbing.

By the end of the day, the students had formed a very visible bond with each other. An atmosphere of comrades-in-arms prevailed, in which the students helped each other at a moment's notice, without any hesitation or judgment.

After dinner we sat around the campfire and discussed how the day unfolded for us. We went around the circle and listened to what each student had to say. Many thoughts and emotions bubbled to the surface. A few tears were shed—the tears that come when the heart begins to crack open. Jerome said, "I'd like to acknowledge how much Jackson has helped me. I don't think I could have made it this far on the course without him."

When it was Jackson's turn to speak, he said, "Something's going on inside me." He struggled to express exactly what he was referring to. "It's good, Man. It's all good," he assured us as he wiped away a few tears with the back of his hand. "I guess I love bossing people around," he said with a big smile. In his own way, he told us how good it felt to be able to help other people.

After the debriefing, I acknowledged how well the students kept their promise not to reveal their identities, other than their names, over the past three days. Now they could talk about who they were in their lives back home, what motivated them to take the COBS course, what their jobs were, their ages, and what they hoped to get from the course. We went around the circle revealing our identities. Only two people chose to withhold that information—Jerome and Jackson, who had become inseparable buddies, their age difference and positions in society notwithstanding.

Just before we headed off to bed, Patricia asked me to reveal my identity by describing my life before teaching for Outward Bound. I briefly summarized my adult life and wrapped up by saying that I was still searching for my life's purpose. I said that I wanted to use my strengths to make a meaningful difference in people's lives by helping empower them to be their best selves. Patricia said, "Well, it looks like you're doing exactly that with us." Heads nodded in agreement. After a long silence, we put out the campfire and went to bed.

On the fourth day, at the students' request, we did more rock climbing in the morning and then took the rest of the day off to write in our journals and do whatever else we wanted. Jerome and Jackson took a short hike together. Each student had a whistle to use if they faced any danger or got lost.

On the fifth day, I designated Mandy as our leader. The thought of leading the group created intense anxiety for her. With constant coaching by me, and with encouragement from the group, Mandy began to feel more secure. I asked Jackson to teach her how to use the map and compass to guide us to our day's destination. The students treated her with kindness and patience. By the time we reached our campsite, Mandy was in full control of her leadership position and did a perfect job with making the dinner and rounding up help with the dishes.

We spent the evening around the campfire reviewing the events of the day and sharing our thoughts and feelings. Mandy confessed that during the first days on the course she had intense cravings for sodas, junk food, and anything sugary, but that she had finally overcome those symptoms of withdrawal and was feeling better than she had in years. We ended the evening singing popular songs and telling ghost stories.

The following day we stayed at our campsite and learned wilderness first aid. The students were eager to learn how to respond to various unanticipated major and minor disasters. I loved teaching these skills, many of which I learned during a wilderness first aid course I took in Boulder, Colorado.

Jerome wanted to know what we would do if someone had a heart attack in the mountains. I think he might have been worried about that possibility, given his age and our strenuous activity. I had felt reassured when I read in the paperwork that he had a full cardiac evaluation before signing up for the OB course. I reminded him of this fact and also let him know that, in the unlikely event of a heart attack, I would radio for help to the OB staff in Crestone and request immediate help with evacuation. I also reassured him that I was trained in CPR.

Besides addressing Jerome's question, I taught the students how to deal with an extensive range of common conditions, including altitude sickness, heat stroke, frostbite, concussions, lacerations, food poisoning, and fractures needing immobilization and evacuation. We jerry-rigged stretchers by using two long poles from young aspen tree trunks that I cut down with my little axe. We threaded the poles through the sleeves of a few of our jackets. The students also learned how to carry an injured person if there was no one else available to help. I had no idea that I would soon be using that technique with a student on the course.

On the following day we slowly hiked along a very steep and arduous switchback trail that wound up the side of a mountain. In the distance we could see the rocky pass we needed to cross in order to get to our designated campsite on the other side.

When we were about 100 feet below the pass, Mandy said she could not keep going. Her fear of heights immobilized her, especially after she glanced down the steep slope we had walked up. "I cannot cross that ridge to the other side. Just looking at it makes me feel sick, like I'm going to vomit or pass out."

No amount of encouragement changed her mind. I had to make a decision about what to do. After a few minutes of reflection, I put down my pack and pulled out the climbing gear. I gave Jackson the rope and asked if he would be comfortable anchoring himself into a boulder at the top of the pass and belaying Mandy up the mountain. He eagerly accepted the task. After clipping Mandy into one end of the rope, Jackson took the rest of the uncoiling rope to the top of the pass and set himself up for the belay.

I pondered what to do about Mandy's backpack. Johnny read my mind and offered to go to the top of the pass, drop his pack, and return to pick up hers.

I asked Patricia to lead the rest of the students over the pass and down the other side, where she would see a large, grassy ledge. I instructed them to wait there for Mandy, Jackson, and me to join them.

Mandy still refused to budge. After my many failed attempts to change her mind, she finally agreed to let me carry her on my back up to the pass. I was uncertain if I could pull this off, given that Mandy was significantly heavier than me.

I put on my harness and clipped myself into the rope, creating an improvised arrangement that included both of us being on belay. I signaled to Jackson to take up the slack.

After Jackson yelled, "ON BELAY," I hoisted Mandy's heavy body diagonally across my back and right shoulder in a fireman's carry.

With sheer willpower and a rush of fear-induced adrenaline, I managed to slowly move along the steep and narrow trail, one step in front of the other, with my heart racing and gasping for air. Mandy whimpered continuously, certain she was going to die.

When we got safely to the top of the pass, I gently lowered Mandy onto solid ground and untied her. After a short crying spell from pent-up tension, Mandy looked down the other side where the students were waiting for us. She said the trail down to them was too steep. Jackson managed to talk her into letting him rappel her down to the less steep area.

When she landed on the grassy ledge, the group clapped and cheered. Mandy got hugs from all her fellow students. She smiled through her tears.

Jackson retrieved my backpack, then climbed back up to the pass and down the other side. The students gave Jackson kudos worthy of a hero. He diverted the focus from himself and moved it back to Mandy. He said in a brotherly way, "Girl, I'm so proud of you. You looked that fearful demon right in the eye. Yes, you did."

After a short rest, we continued to drop down into a stunningly beautiful bowl-shaped basin, created by a former glacier. We headed over to the alpine lake with pristine, turquoise-colored water and set up camp.

Around the campfire that night, many of the students, both the men and the women, got choked up as they shared their feelings of joy, accomplishment, and the ability to overcome their fears. They were not only proud of themselves, but proud of their fellow team members. I had to wipe away a few tears. The encouragement and compassion the students showed each other moved me deeply.

Surprisingly, they showed empathy for me as well, acknowledging how scary it must have been to carry Mandy up the steep slope to the top of the pass. I believed in being transparent with the students and admitted that I had some scary thoughts going up to the pass.

A long moment of silent reflection occurred spontaneously. Johnny, a strikingly handsome 26-year-old bartender in search of a more meaningful path in life, broke the silence. "Mandy's amazing act of courage in facing her fear inspires me and gives me the courage to make a confession to the group: I am gay. I just recently came out of the closet to my parents. My father practically disowned me."

Jackson spoke up, "Man, you think we didn't know? Does it really matter to us who you have sex with? We love you, brother. You're just fine the way you are." Heads nodded in agreement while the tears flowed. As though on cue, everyone stood up and walked over to Johnny to give him a big, group hug.

After another long silence as we stared at the flames of the campfire, Luc spoke up, saying he didn't realize how good it felt to be part of a team and to help each other out. He said he was thinking about joining the French Foreign Legion so he could fight with other soldiers for justice and freedom from tyranny. It wasn't clear whether he was serious or being his usual humorous self.

Allison and Cindy, the young women who had initially wanted to quit and go home, expressed to the group their surprise that they had been able to endure thus far the many challenges on the course. They began to understand that they were capable of far more than they ever imagined. They both admitted that they were proud of themselves and couldn't wait to tell their family and friends about the course.

Cindy marveled that she could carry everything she needed on her back. She said that when she got home, she was going to donate at least half her wardrobe to Goodwill. She confessed how freeing it was not to use makeup on the course and to just be herself.

Tim, a quiet and reserved 18-year-old young man, always observing and attentive, spoke next. "I haven't talked much on this course. I'm not very outgoing. But, I'm really inspired by everyone's willingness to be open with each other and share on such a deep and heartfelt level. So, I want to share with you something about myself. I come from a blue-collar, working class family living just above the poverty level. I worked hard in school and got a merit scholarship to attend Stanford in the fall. I also got a monetary award for graduating from high school near the top of my class. I used that award money to pay for this Outward Bound course. This has been the best investment I could have made. I have learned so much from all of you. Thank you." Tim choked up as he spoke.

I was surprised when I looked at my watch. It was way past our usual bedtime.

As the days progressed, we moved higher up the side of a massive mountain, called Kit Carson. Our gradual ascent in stages, on circuitous routes far off the beaten path, allowed the students to become well acclimatized to the altitude and get into shape physically. No one showed any signs of altitude sickness.

Several days into the course, we came to a large snow and ice field, the remnant of a former glacier. On this icy expanse I taught the students a new set of skills that included roping up as a team, kicking with each step to secure one's footing in the crusty snow, and skillfully using their ice axes. We made large switchbacks as we ascended the slope. The part of the day the students enjoyed the most was glissading down the slope, using their bodies as a toboggan, and then self-arresting by slamming the pick of the ice axe into the hardened snow. I heard lots of squeals of delight.

Luc made about a dozen snowballs the size of baseballs and stacked them in his backpack. When I asked him what he was doing, he said he was going to use the snowballs to clean himself. He said he didn't like using "toilet paper plants" and smooth little stones to clean his behind, and then having to sanitize his hands afterwards. He said using snowballs was more hygienic and had no impact on the environment. Luc had a great idea but by the time we reached our campsite, the snowballs had melted in his pack. Fortunately, Luc had a good sense of humor.

The following day we hiked along a stream with a series of waterfalls to a pristine alpine lake at around 11,000 feet. A palpable feeling of awe and reverence came over all of us as we surveyed our spectacular surroundings, with views of Kit Carson Mountain, Crestone Needle, and Crestone Peak looming over us like giant sentinels. I suggested that we put down our packs and sit in silence for a few minutes to take in the wondrous scene surrounding us.

Our meditative session ended abruptly when we heard a loud clatter and sounds of falling rocks. We looked up and saw a large bighorn sheep descending a rocky area above us. The magnificent animal stopped on a flat, oblong granite rock and stared at us. We stared back, mesmerized by the ram's elegant stature, with his massive brown horns curled around the sides of his face.

We spent the rest of the day exploring the area, setting up camp, followed by a long discussion regarding the next day's ascent of Kit Carson Mountain. I assured the group that they had learned to work well as a team and that they had the stamina and the altitude adaptation to reach the summit. The most difficult part of the climb would be the loose rocks and patches of snow and ice that could cause us to slip and fall, especially on the descent.

Patricia asked me what I personally did to deal with fear and anxiety. I demonstrated a simple breathing technique, which involved prolonging the length of the inhalations and exhalations. Slowing the breath calms the nervous system, a fact well known by gurus all the way back to ancient times.

To test out the system, I asked the students to think of a frightening scene in front of them. First I asked them to breathe hard and fast with shallow breaths as they contemplated the imaginary scene. Then I asked them to change to deep, slow breathing and see what happens. I also shared with them a special kind of yogic breathing called *pranayama*.

The students continued to ask for more tips for controlling their fear. The most useful one I could think of was to put one's full focus on the present moment—in this case, it would mean focusing on putting one foot in front of the other.

I asked Mandy if she would like to stay in camp and not participate in the summit climb. To everyone's utter amazement, Mandy said she wanted to go with us to the top. She said she was tired of living in fear. The group praised her decision.

We unanimously decided not to have a fire circle and, instead, go straight to bed.

I woke the students up at four o'clock the next morning. Getting up in the dark would normally be challenging, but the students were so full of anticipatory excitement, they hardly slept during the night. With their headlamps on, they got dressed, filled their water bottles, and got their gear ready to go. I made coffee for everyone.

In our daypacks we put plenty of snacks and two water bottles, sunglasses, warm clothing, our map and compass, and our cameras. I carried the rope and first aid kit. We donned our helmets and our bright yellow Helly Hansen rain gear in case of inclement weather. Rainstorms frequently occurred in the mountains in the afternoon, and sometimes snowstorms occurred in early spring at that altitude.

By five o'clock we were en route to the summit, 3,000 feet above us.

We paired up so that each person had a buddy. Mandy asked to pair with me.

I resumed my role as leader of the day, setting a slow but steady pace. I asked Jackson to walk in the rear and make sure no one had a problem that needed addressing.

In complete silence, we walked with our headlamps illuminating the well-traveled switchbacks. When the sun rose on the horizon, we stopped to eat our power bar breakfast, hydrate, and check in with each other. The students were enthusiastic and slightly apprehensive at the same time.

After a couple of hours we reached the steep, slippery section with lots of loose rocks. As we ascended, I often had to hold Mandy's hand or arm to steady her gait. She had made a commitment not to look down the mountain and just keep her eyes looking forward. She was terrified, but determined to keep going. I reminded her to practice the special breathing technique.

I asked the students to stay close together so that if someone dislodged a rock we would know immediately and take action to get out of its way before it gained momentum.

We reached the summit just before noon. After group hugs and lots of jubilation, we sat down and once more I requested a moment of silence as we took in the spectacular views from the top of Kit Carson Mountain. We could see the summits of all the surrounding mountains, and we even caught a glimpse of the Great Sand Dunes.

After we ate our lunches, I reminded the students of the need to get off the mountain before the predictable afternoon mountain rain and possible lightning storm set in, which would make our descent very precarious.

The descent was much more difficult and tedious than the ascent. Each step had to be placed with one's fully focused attention in order not to slip. I told the students that what they were doing was a form of mindfulness meditation. Barely a word was spoken.

I made sure that if someone dislodged a rock, they had to loudly yell, "ROCK," so that the people below could get out of the way. There were times when Mandy was so frightened, she sat down and inched her way down on her bottom.

In the late afternoon, just as we reached the safety of the switchbacks, the sky darkened and let loose torrents of hard driving rain. We arrived back at our campsite in the late afternoon, after the downpour had subsided. The students suggested that we all help out to make an early dinner and then go to bed. Most of them were too tired to participate in our usual fire circle debriefing.

The next morning the students were in a celebratory mood, but their bodies looked stiff as they walked around the campsite. I offered to teach them some simple yoga poses, like the downward facing dog, that would help stretch out their muscles and loosen up their joints. This little class was so popular that some of the students did a shortened version every morning for the rest of the expedition.

As we ate our breakfast someone pointed out three deer among the trees. They were looking at us as though they were curious about what we were doing. After breakfast we had a short debriefing of our summit climb. The students repeatedly praised Mandy for her bravery. The only regret they expressed was that they forgot to take pictures with their cameras because, as one person said, "We were deeply focused on the present moment."

The rest of the day the students spent swimming, unabashedly naked, in the pristine alpine lake, taking little walks in the surrounding forest, and writing in their journals. Tim and Johnny walked above timberline to look for more bighorn sheep. Instead, they saw lots of pika, small rodent-like mammals with rounded ears that live in wind-swept alpine areas. They make high-pitched squeaky sounds to alert others of predators. The pika share their habitats with marmots, which are the size of a large, furry cat. Tim and Johnny discussed the possibility of trying to catch one of the marmots sitting on a rock in the sun. They both were starved for fresh meat.

At fire circle that evening, I spoke about mountains being a metaphor for the unavoidable challenges we all face throughout our lives. "You will inevitably encounter lots of scary mountains in the form of health challenges, relationship problems, financial hardship, and anything else that seems daunting and overwhelming. You can think back on the time you climbed these mountains in spite of your fears and the limiting beliefs about what you were capable of doing."

I went on to say, "Watching all of you on this course reminds me of my own journey overcoming my inner demons and distorted views of myself. I climbed some very high mountains in South America. Those mountains were symbols for me. Like you are doing on this course, I learned a lot about myself." The students asked if I would talk more about my life. They asked me endless questions. We talked far into the night, long after the campfire had died out. The chilly night air eventually made us retreat into our tents.

We spent the following two days wending our way through forests on unmarked trails until we reached the base of Crestone Needle, yet another one of the many 14,000-foot mountains in the area. The group, including Mandy, expertly navigated the seemingly endless gully, full of loose rocks and patches of snow and ice. Some of the students shouted for joy when we reached the summit. We stood in silent reverence for at least 15 minutes as we soaked in the grandeur.

While we ate our lunch, the sky suddenly became dark and the temperature dropped precipitously. We cut our lunch short and immediately headed down the mountain. As before, the descent was significantly more difficult than the climb up the gully. We had to be mindful of every step we took. When we had descended halfway down the gully, snow began to fall, propelled by fierce winds. We found a small, flat area behind a large boulder, where we huddled together until the wind subsided and the visibility improved.

We arrived back at camp cold and tired. Patricia shook uncontrollably and showed signs of hypothermia. Jerome offered to make hot soup for her. I asked her tent mate, Mandy, to help Patricia warm up by zipping their sleeping bags together, and for Mandy to hold Patricia in a full body embrace while in the sleeping bags. With the hot soup and the heat from Mandy's body, Patricia recovered quickly.

While looking for wood to make a campfire that night, I saw two piles of bear poop near our tents, as well as the tracks of bighorn sheep.

At the fire circle, after the students checked in with how they were doing, I suggested that they tell a short story about their prior lives. Jerome spoke first. He said that he was finally ready to reveal to the group who he was in his former life. When he said he was a 60-year-old, recently retired professor of math at MIT, the students looked stunned. He said that he had spent very little time in his life doing outdoor activities, had never been in the wilderness, and had never carried a backpack. He said that this OB course was one of the most physically and psychologically challenging experiences he had ever had.

The students responded to Jerome's revelation in amazement that he had the courage to come on this course with mostly young people. They praised him for not giving up during the times he felt he couldn't go on. Johnny said, "Professor, I'm sure it took a lot of guts to sign up for this expedition."

During Jerome's revelations, he expressed once again how deeply grateful he was to Jackson for all of his help and encouragement. He said he hoped that the two of them would remain lifelong friends.

When it was Jackson's turn to reveal his identity, he described his chaotic and gut-wrenching life as a young child with abusive, alcoholic, and impoverished parents. The group listened spellbound as he described with unfiltered honesty the antisocial activities he had engaged in and all the harm he had done to people and property.

Jackson said that he hadn't wanted to talk earlier about his past because he felt he would be judged harshly and not given a chance. He said how grateful he was to the judge who saw his potential and offered an alternative to jail.

During the course, Jackson had an epiphany. He said, "I didn't realize how good it feels to be a leader and help people out. I really want to help the kids in my neighborhood get out of gang life and do something meaningful. Someday I'm gonna open my own version of an Outward Bound school and offer courses for gang members who want a different life for themselves. It doesn't hurt to dream big."

Jerome spoke up and said that he would like to help him get through high school and college and was willing to personally tutor him if necessary. He said he would also help him strategize and find the funding to open his own outdoor school.

The next morning, after breakfast, we packed up our gear, making sure to leave the campsite as pristine as we found it, with no trace of our presence. We had a long hike ahead of us into a neighboring valley, where we would set up camp next to a fast-flowing creek.

During one of our rest stops en route, I introduced the students to a part of the OB course called the "Solo," in which each student remains completely alone for three days, making no contact with anyone unless there was an emergency. The students could take with them in their backpacks a tarp, sleeping bag and pad, a water bottle, iodine tablets, toiletries, warm clothes, rain gear, a headlamp, a whistle, a journal, and a pen—and that's it. No food.

"What? We're going to be all alone and fast for three days? No food? You've got to be kidding!" Allison was incredulous. For the rest of the hike I heard anxiety-laden speculation among the students about the upcoming Solo.

After we arrived at our campsite beside the creek, we ate dinner and then sat around the campfire to discuss the Solo experience. To my surprise, Jackson seemed the most fearful. He was afraid of being alone in total silence. He said he had never been totally alone in his entire life. He asked what he should do if a bear came to his campsite. I reassured him that there would be no food to attract the bears.

Mandy was the one most afraid of going without food for three days and wondered if she could do it. She had never gone more than a few hours without eating.

Tim asked what purpose the Solo served. I shared with him and the others my view of the Solo as a time to become inwardly still and reflect on one's life, without distractions.

The students wrote in their journals the topics I suggested for them to ponder: What have you learned about yourself from this course? What inner strengths did you discover you have? What would you like to change about yourself? What is meaningful to you and makes you feel good about yourself? Do you see a purpose for your life? What would you like to accomplish in the future?

The next morning, after their coffee, the students prepared for their departure. One by one, I took them to their designated sites next to the creek. No one could see each other. On the trail I made a cairn with a little pile of rocks to indicate where I needed to turn to locate each student's Solo site. I let the students know that if they needed my help, and it wasn't an emergency, they could leave a note under one of the stones. If they had an emergency, I instructed them to blow their whistle three times and then repeat the series.

After I had placed all nine students on their Solo sites, I returned to the campsite. I decided that I would do my own modified version of a Solo as an act of solidarity with my students, including fasting. I got out my journal and spent much of the day writing about the OB course. I also followed the advice I gave to my students and wrote what I learned about myself and where my strengths and weaknesses lay. And, as I often did, I pondered the ultimate purpose of my life.

In the middle of the day and again in the late afternoon I checked up on each student. I silently approached their sites and stood within viewing distance to make sure they were all right.

Back at the campsite, I set up my pad and sleeping bag on a little patch of grass. I left my tent in my backpack because I preferred sleeping outside under the stars.

Before going to bed, I confess that I lowered one of the food bags suspended from the branch of a nearby tree and took out the jar of honey. I took my special hand-carved wooden spoon and dipped it into the honey jar, then slowly and blissfully licked the honey off the spoon, feeling very guilty about my behavior.

A few drops of honey fell onto the end of my sleeping bag. I licked the area, and then wiped it with a damp cloth. I put the jar back in the food bag and re-suspended it from the branch. Then I brushed my teeth, rinsed my mouth, and crawled inside my sleeping bag.

In the early morning, while sleeping, I felt something moving the end of my sleeping bag where my feet were. I opened my eyes and lifted my head. In the pale moonlight I saw a young black bear licking the place where I had spilled a few drops of honey. He looked up at me nonchalantly, and then he turned around and slowly lumbered toward the creek.

The three days passed quickly. I picked up the students in the afternoon of the third day and walked with them back to camp. We spent the rest of the afternoon and evening around the campfire, sharing our intimate thoughts, feelings, aspirations, and intentions.

Some people read to the group what they wrote in their journals. Mandy filled her journal with mouth-watering recipes along with her thoughts about how she wanted to channel her food addiction problems into running a restaurant and making exceptional culinary experiences for the customers. She learned from the course that she was braver than she realized and could overcome her fears—including the fear of starting her own business.

On the subject of food addiction, I confessed to the group what I did with the honey and the subsequent encounter with the young bear that licked my sleeping bag. The group thought the story was hilarious. Johnny said he was relieved to hear that I wasn't perfect.

Jerome said that whatever he decided to do in his retirement, it had to be something meaningful that made a difference in young people's lives. He made a commitment in his mind to help Jackson eventually achieve his dream.

Jackson said that the first day of the Solo was Hell. Being totally alone in complete silence was one of the scariest things he had ever done. He was proud of himself that he didn't blow the whistle and was able to breathe through his fear. He said to himself, "If Mandy can make it to the top of two mountains, then I can make it through these three days."

Jackson had big plans for himself, his family, and his community. His first goal was to write a personal letter to the judge, thanking him for believing that he had the potential to turn his life around.

Every one of the students had a powerful experience being alone for three days on the Solo. I knew the bond between them was so strong that some of the friendships would continue long after they returned home.

The course was rapidly coming to a close. On the two-day hike out of the wilderness, we passed a sheep ranch. Johnny made an outlandish request. He said he was starved for some good meat and suggested we ask the rancher to sell us two legs of lamb we could roast over the fire. The idea sounded intriguing. I found a $20 bill in my pocket and hoped it would be enough to get what we wanted. The rancher agreed to butcher a lamb and sell us two legs. I asked the students to watch the rancher butcher the lamb so that they would know exactly what's involved when eating meat. For some, the process was eye opening and thought provoking. For others it was repulsive to watch the lamb being slaughtered. Patricia said she was never going to eat meat again.

We roasted the lamb meat over our campfire. Everyone ate a piece of the lamb, including Patricia.

It was our last evening together before we said goodbye to each other the next day. At the time of departure, there wasn't a dry eye to be found. There were long, heartfelt hugs and last-minute exchanges of addresses and phone numbers and promises to stay in touch.

I waved as the bus drove away. Strong emotions filled me with a mixture of both exhilaration and tearful sadness. I felt like a mother, waving goodbye to her children as they go off to college after graduating from high school.

It wasn't long before I began receiving letters from the parents of the students. Cindy's mother wrote a letter that expressed a common reaction that I heard repeatedly from other parents: "What did you do to my daughter? She's a different person—very grown up. She takes responsibility for her actions. She helps around the house and is polite. She actually treats her family with respect!!!! She's even talking about starting her own charitable business repurposing her used clothing to help poor people."

The OB course was not just about wilderness survival and climbing big mountains. Those activities were vehicles for personal growth, learning how to work as a team supporting each other, developing empathy and compassion, discovering what one is capable of doing and how to make a difference in the world.

I taught for the Colorado Outward Bound School for three summers, from 1977 through 1979. I loved teaching those courses. It was deeply fulfilling to be able to make a significant difference in people's lives—and in such a beautiful setting. I often wondered if teaching experiential education was my true purpose in life.

Chapter 32

BURIED ALIVE

I HELD JOE NOLD IN HIGH REGARD and followed his advice to the letter. He asked me to get trained as an emergency medical technician (EMT) so I could be prepared for dealing with any accidents that might occur while teaching courses in the wilderness. I found the idea intriguing and eagerly pursued the necessary steps to apply for the training.

The master's program did not require very much time or effort beyond reading several books about education, participating in roundtable discussions, keeping a detailed journal, and debriefing with Joe, along with writing a few papers. I had adequate time to focus on the training required in becoming an EMT.

It usually takes about six months to complete the 180 hours of training. After that, the student takes a state certification test. An EMT can provide emergency treatment in ambulances and many other venues. I had no intention of working exclusively as an EMT; I simply wanted to have the skills in case I faced an emergency while in the wilderness.

I found the on-the-job aspect of the training thrilling. I followed the emergency room doctors throughout the day for one week at two major hospitals in Denver and one in Boulder. I got paired up with some excellent doctors who explained to me much of what they were doing—the procedures, why they ordered certain tests, what the results meant, the pathology that had made the patient sick, the prognosis, and the referrals for aftercare.

The patients seemed to enjoy listening to the doctor talking to me about their cases. One of the doctors even let me stitch up a patient's cut leg, with the patient's consent and under his guidance.

While the patients waited to get evaluated by the doctor, I spent time talking with them and asking about their symptoms. I found this aspect of my training just as rewarding as watching the doctor's evaluations and treatments.

I wished I could go every day to shadow the ER doctor. I was sorry when the course ended. I longed for more ER experiences.

Upon certification, I joined the Rocky Mountain Search and Rescue Group, which searched for lost, injured, or dead climbers in the surrounding mountains. My experience with rescuing climbers was limited because I was only available on certain weekends.

One weekend I had my own unanticipated search and rescue experience.

On a sunny winter day, I drove with one of my friends from Boulder to the top of a high mountain pass in the Colorado Rockies. We parked our car and headed off into the wilderness with our skis strapped to our backpacks. Our spirits were high.

A few days prior, this particular area of the Rockies had seen a heavy snowstorm that dumped an estimated two feet of snow in the mountains. On the day of our outing, the weather had warmed to well above freezing. There wasn't a cloud in the sky.

We carefully picked our way down the mountain on a rocky

ridge-like outcropping until we came to an area where the angle of the slope was not as steep and appeared safe for backcountry skiing. We stepped onto the snowy slope. While breaking trail in search of a spot conducive for putting on our skis, I noticed that the snow felt hollow under my feet. I heard "whumping" sounds, indicating that the snow was settling, arousing in me a sense of foreboding.

I told Jamey that I feared we might cause an avalanche, given the angle of the slope and the freshly fallen snow that had not totally consolidated. I knew that sunny days after a snowstorm could cause some of the snow on the surface to melt and trickle down through the snow. During the cold nights, the water freezes, creating a sliding surface. I discussed my concerns with Jamey. He agreed that we should go back to the rocky outcropping and walk down until the slope became less steep.

Jamey had already taken off his pack and untied his skis when I expressed my concern. Instead of waiting for him while he worked with his gear, I turned around and began walking back to the ridge. Not long after I stepped onto the rocky ground, I heard a terrifying rumbling sound that reverberated throughout the narrow valley. I turned and watched in horror as the entire slope cracked several yards above where Jamey stood. Within seconds, Jamey disappeared in a huge cloud of snow and ice that roared down the mountain like a raging river. The avalanche felt like it lasted an eternity, but in reality it probably was only a few minutes. I had lost all sense of time as I watched in a state of primordial terror and awe.

After the avalanche completed its descent, total silence enveloped the valley. Big blocks of compacted snow and ice the size of small cars lay at the base of the slope. With my heart racing, I carefully picked my way over to the area where the avalanche had swept Jamey away. I removed the baskets from my ski poles and poked them into the snow, probing every couple of feet, hoping to find Jamey's body.

I walked and probed an area the size of a football field, zigzagging back and forth, beginning where Jamey first disappeared, all the way to where the avalanche ended. My eyes grew weary from straining to spot something other than the various shades of white. Over and over I cried out my friend's name in desperation. "Jamey! Jamey! Jamey! God, help me find Jamey!" The mountain responded to my cries with deathly silence.

I looked at my watch and saw that it was already three o'clock. I had searched in vain for Jamey for what felt like hours. The winter sun would set in less than three hours. Even with my headlamp, it would be hard to find my way to the paved road after dark, given that there was no trail.

I had to make a gut-wrenching decision. Do I leave now to save my own life? Or do I keep looking fruitlessly for Jamey into the night and risk freezing to death? I felt ripped apart inside, having to make such a horrible choice. I decided that risking my life would be of no benefit to Jamey and would cause deep pain for my family.

I kneeled down and said a prayer for Jamey. As I sobbed, I said out loud, "I'm so terribly sorry to leave you, Jamey." With a heavy heart, I stood up and walked down to a more level place where I could put on my backcountry skis. As I untied the skis from my backpack, I saw something out of the corner of my eye—something that was not white. Off in the distance a pink-colored object protruded from the snow. I decided to see what it was. As I got closer, I could clearly see the shape of a hand and forearm. I screamed, "JAMEY!" His fingers moved. I held his hand and yelled, "I'm here, Jamey. Hang on. I'm going to dig you out."

My hands could not even make a dent in the hard-packed snow. I took the end of one of my skis and used it like a shovel. Slowly, and with great effort, I cleared the hard snow away from Jamey's head. He had instinctively placed his gloved hand over his mouth, keeping the snow from suffocating him and giving him a pocket of air to breathe. He was in a stupor and barely responsive. He looked at me and, in a tiny, barely audible voice, said, "Thank you, Erica."

After an exhausting hour of digging, Jamey's chest and arms were free. The rest of his body took much less time to dig out. At last, Jamey extricated himself from his tomb. He had lost his backpack, skis, poles, camera, hat, and one of his gloves in the avalanche. I hugged him tightly while his whole body shook in my arms. His clothes were wet. I gave him my hat and gloves and insisted that he drink the rest of my water.

We had to start moving right away, not only to help warm Jamey's body, but also to avoid getting lost after the sun went down. I put on my skis and packed down the snow with each step so that Jamey would not sink into the snow as he walked behind me. In spite of my efforts, he still sank, sometimes up to his knees, as we plowed through the willows along the stream we followed. We made painfully slow progress.

We had less than an hour before the sun would go below the horizon. Jamey sat down on a log and said he couldn't go any farther. I talked to him firmly, using my Outward Bound instructor voice, "Jamey, you just have to keep walking no matter how tired you are. Get up now. We have to keep moving." I knew he was severely hypothermic from his wet clothes, beaten and battered from the fall, and running on empty. He would have to rely on pure willpower to get out of here alive. Once again, I took on the role of drill sergeant and insisted that he keep walking. "I'm not going to let you die out here, Jamey."

He trudged on, but stopped again saying he had to pee. He walked away from me behind some trees. When he hadn't returned after a few minutes, I followed his footsteps into a wooded area and found him with his arms around a tree, softly crying in gratitude for being alive.

After enormous effort, we managed to make it back to Boulder. Although we both continued to enjoy our respective backcountry adventures, Jamey had nightmares about being entombed in snow and slowly suffocating to death, while I had nightmares about trying to rescue people in distress. I had no idea that I would someday take on this role in real life.

Chapter 33

STANFORD INTERVIEW

WHILE IN BOULDER, I encountered several first-year medical students from CU on my weekend forays into the Rocky Mountains. They seemed very excited about their training. I thought about what my father said when he urged me to consider becoming a doctor, but I dismissed the idea as unrealistic.

Midway through the master's program, after I had completed my EMT training, I decided to take some science courses on the side. Antioch College had waived all my science requirements due to my high scores on the tests given at the time of admission.

Now, over a decade later, I felt I had missed out. I hungered to explore the sciences, especially after learning about anatomy and physiology in my EMT training. I enrolled in an AP Biology 101 class for freshmen at CU, not realizing that it was primarily for pre-med students.

I had considered the possibility of becoming a doctor at various times while in the Peace Corps, but dismissed the idea, thinking that one had to have extraordinarily high intelligence to pursue this route.

I thought about the Swiss doctors in my family—my grandfather, who had served an entire town in northern Switzerland, and my brilliant Uncle Ernst, with whom I spent a summer after graduating from college. He made a big impression on me. I admired his ability to cure the "incurables" who came from many countries to receive his treatments. His patients told me he was a true genius. No one had ever referred to me as a true genius, so I never seriously considered becoming a doctor.

When I started taking science classes at the University of Colorado, I observed my young pre-med classmates. They did not appear to be extraordinarily brilliant. I noticed that what they all had in common was a tremendous capacity for memorization and getting high grades on standardized tests. Perhaps the students did indeed have the capacity for critical thinking and asking questions about what they were learning—but the kind of teaching they got did not encourage that skill.

> *These kids will be our future doctors? Hmm. Well, if they can do it, I certainly can too! I'm good at memorizing. I remember being commended by my first-grade teacher in England for my ability to recite long poems from memory—even ones that I didn't understand.*

A wave of excitement washed over me as I realized I could indeed become a doctor without having to be a genius, like my Uncle Ernst in Switzerland. A slumbering force deep within me awakened with the clear recognition that I had finally stumbled upon the path that would lead me to my true calling in life.

On an early morning walk by myself in the mountains, I stopped at the edge of a small alpine lake and looked up at the sky. I yelled for joy, "I've found my purpose! I'm going to be a doctor. Thank you, God!"

When I got back to my little room, I took my dictionary off the shelf and looked up the word "doctor." I learned that the word was derived from the Latin word *docere*, which means, "to teach."

Suddenly, the pieces of my life's puzzle were starting to fit together and form a distinct picture.

Some of those pieces included my love of teaching, especially when the teaching involved something that would empower people and ultimately enhance their lives. Other pieces related to my fascination with the human body and its workings, an intense curiosity about life, and an insatiable love of learning. Even when I was much younger, I had an interest in trying to solve health-related problems, including my own. I got a vicarious thrill when I could do something that made people feel better.

Doctoring could also be a vehicle for expressing my love and compassion for people, just as teaching had been for me when I taught Navajo children in the fourth grade on the reservation.

With focus and determination, I signed up for every pre-med course I could squeeze into my schedule while finishing the final requirements for my master's degree.

One day after class, my chemistry teacher advised me to talk to a guidance counselor about my desire to become a doctor, implying that I might be too old for medical school.

The guidance counselor was a serious-looking, silver-haired man. "You're here to discuss the possibility of applying for medical school. Is that correct, Miss Elliott?"

"Yes. That's correct." I told him that I was thinking of applying to two or three schools and wondered if he had any advice for me.

He did indeed have advice for me. He said, "Although you have an impressive file, I have concluded nevertheless that it would be best for you to let go of the idea of going into medicine." He thought I should consider becoming a teacher or a professor because it was obvious how much I enjoyed teaching. He said that medicine was not the right career choice for me and that I'd be wasting my time and money applying to medical school.

I stood in front of the guidance counselor in silence, the wind knocked out of me. It took a few seconds before I could regain my breath. "Why do you say that?"

"I'm trying to do you a favor and spare you disappointment and the costly expenses of the application process." He said my file revealed several items against me.

"First of all, you're a woman. Women have a harder time getting into medical school. Second, you're 29 years old. That's too old to be thinking about pre-med and all that's involved in getting into medical school. You'd be in your *thirties* when you were ready to apply. And third, you have a liberal arts background, not science. You have done nothing in your past that is related to medicine, except the EMT certification course. Not good," he said gravely.

As he looked at my résumé, he said, "You've been a schoolteacher on the Navajo Reservation, a Peace Corps volunteer in South America, a mountaineer, and an Outward Bound instructor, and you just recently completed your master's degree in outdoor experiential education. The admissions people at the medical schools will wonder if you have what it takes to stick to one thing.

"I don't think you have a chance at getting accepted into any medical school. I'm sorry. I'm just being honest with you."

My answer was polite, but with a tinge of defiance. "Never underestimate the power of a vision, Sir. I *know* that medicine is my path in life. I believe it's my destiny. It just took me a while to realize it. I'll let you know what happens with the applications."

The guidance counselor's discouraging remarks made me more

determined than ever. I applied right away to take the medical college admission test, or MCAT, even though at that point, I'd only taken one year of pre-med courses. I still lacked half of the requirements, including the major subjects like advanced chemistry, biochemistry, and physics.

Pre-med students were supposed to finish the two years of pre-med requirements and then wait until the next MCAT test was offered. If their scores were decent, they would apply to medical schools, followed by a year of waiting to see if they were accepted for the following fall.

I didn't want to wait that long. If I followed the rules, I'd be two years older by the time I applied. Hadn't the guidance counselor said I was already too old at 29?

The MCAT was a daunting test that took almost eight hours to complete. Aspiring young doctors packed the auditorium. Half the questions pertained to courses I had not yet taken, so I had no choice but to guess the answers to those questions.

By some stroke of luck, I scored the national average on the MCAT test—probably not high enough to get into a top-notch medical school. But I wasn't going to let my mediocre scores deter me from applying to Stanford, the University of Colorado, and Dartmouth medical schools.

I waited impatiently for a response.

Then an unexpected phone call came. Fortunately, I was home in my cramped little room. Those were the days before answering machines.

A voice said, "Hello. My name is Richard, and I'm calling from the Stanford Admissions office. Is this Erica Elliott?" He informed me that Stanford wanted to give me an interview. He proposed a date and time when I could meet with the admissions people on campus.

"Oh my God! Thank you. That's such good news. But wait. Um. Richard, I just came back from the Peace Corps last year and don't have the money to fly out there for the interview. I have almost no savings. Can you fly out and do the interview here in Boulder?"

The silence on the other end of the phone made me wonder if I'd said something wrong. My thoughts raced around, searching for what to say next.

"Listen, Richard, I could give you an experience you would never forget. If you came out here, we could cross-country ski together into the backcountry in the Colorado Rocky Mountains. You would get to see some of the most beautiful mountain scenery in the world."

I reassured him that he would be in good hands with me. I reminded him that I had been an Outward Bound instructor and had taught dozens of students.

"I could teach you how to navigate on cross-country skis. It's quite easy. Just like walking. I have an extra set of skis and poles I could loan you and then we could rent a pair of boots for you. You would only need to bring warm clothes. I would pack a picnic lunch for both of us. We could sit on a log or some rocky outcropping and eat our lunch in the sun while you interview me. What do you think of that idea?" I took a deep breath.

"Um. Well. Hmm. Let's see. Uh. I'll get back with you after I talk to the head of Admissions."

I excitedly told one of my pre-med classmates about the call from the Stanford Admissions office. He was appalled at what I had proposed. "You did what?! Are you out of your mind?" He explained emphatically how I was supposed to act if I was ever offered another interview, adding, "And I advise you to buy a nice dress, get your hair done, and do whatever it takes to look good when you fly out for the interview."

My classmate predicted Richard would never call back and that I had lost my chance at getting into Stanford. He advised me to play by the rules next time and simply borrow the money to fly to the interviews.

> *Damn! I should have played by the rules—even if I don't know what the rules are. I blew it.*

A week later, Richard called back. He had spoken to the head of Admissions about my request. "Because you are one of the most unusual candidates to apply to Stanford Medical School, I got the go-ahead to interview you in Boulder, Colorado." We set up a time and date to meet.

Richard rented a car at the Denver airport and met me in Boulder with his backpack. He seemed quite excited to have the opportunity to conduct the interview on skis, surrounded by magnificent, jagged peaks on a sunny day in early spring. His voice brimmed with animation and anticipation.

We drove to Rocky Mountain National Park and found a trail with freshly fallen snow. Richard had done a little downhill skiing in the past and had always wanted to try cross-country skiing. He willingly accepted some basic instruction from me. It didn't take long for him to feel at ease on the skinny skis.

As we glided along the trail, Richard said that I had the distinction of having the lowest MCAT scores of anyone Stanford had ever interviewed.

"Should I be proud of that?" I laughed. I confessed to him how pleasantly surprised I was at scoring the national average since I had guessed on half the test questions, unfamiliar as I was with half of the required pre-med course content.

Richard said that the reason the medical school wanted to interview me was because of the out-of-the-ordinary life I had led, my 4.0 grade point average, and especially the letters of recommendation from my professors. One of them had written that I would provide refreshing "leavening" to any school I attended. I wondered what he meant by "leavening" and if that word had other meanings besides making bread rise.

Richard said Stanford liked to include a small percentage of unusual people as part of its student body, people who think "out of the box" and can offer new perspectives.

His voice became serious. "The Admissions department would like to make you an offer. We think you'd be an excellent candidate for our medical school. However, we cannot accept your current MCAT scores. We'd like you to repeat the MCAT test *after* you've completed all the pre-med courses. If you get a score within the top ten percent, then we'll offer you a full four-year scholarship, all expenses paid."

I thanked him for his generous offer and told him I'd think it over. I was in such a hurry to move forward and start my medical studies that, as grand as his offer was, it was still conditional and meant waiting an extra year or more.

Richard told me this interview was the most memorable one he'd ever conducted.

The next day I got a letter from Dartmouth Medical School saying that I was rejected this time around because I had not finished all my pre-med requirements. They suggested I reapply in a year when I had completed all the courses.

A few days later, I got a call from the Admissions department at the University of Colorado requesting an interview. I drove to Denver for the meeting, wearing a dress and high-heeled shoes I had borrowed for the occasion, along with some eyeliner and earrings, and with freshly washed hair. I felt excited and nervous, like I was going to the prom. I just hoped I didn't sprain my ankles in the shoes I wore.

The director of Admissions, a white-haired physician with a kind face, grilled me about why I wanted to be a doctor and why it had taken me so long to make up my mind to pursue medicine.

Toward the end of the long interrogation, the director leaned forward, looking straight into my eyes. Speaking slowly, enunciating each word, he asked, "How do we know you're going to stick with medicine? How do we know you won't move on to something else after you finish your medical training? You've already lived a lifetime with all your various pursuits. Is medical school just one more feather in your cap?"

"Sir, I've come to realize that being a doctor is my real calling. It's my destiny. It's what I'm supposed to be doing with my life. I needed to have a full life before going into medicine. I know that medicine will require all my dedication and energy once I step onto that path. If I had gone straight into medical school right after college, I wouldn't have known anything about life. And besides, I would have been too immature to be a doctor. I know I might seem like an unlikely candidate for medical school, but I promise you that someday you will be proud of me."

The Admissions director sat back in his chair and grinned. He said that the University of Colorado Medical School had already decided to accept me into the next year's program, right after I finished up all my pre-med requirements. He assured me there would be no loss of time waiting. And I would not have to repeat the MCAT test.

Pushing my luck, I told him I had been in the Peace Corps recently and had no money to pay for tuition. He said he was aware of my finances and had already made arrangements for me to receive a full scholarship for the first two years of medical school. The National Health Service Corps would pay for the last two years. In exchange, I would have to serve two years in an underserved area upon the completion of my medical training.

The CU School of Medicine had offered me a good deal, I reckoned. The high cost of my medical education would be covered. And there would be no need to reapply after I finished the premed requirements and take the MCAT a second time, all the while getting older, and risking not scoring in the top ten percent—as required for acceptance into Stanford.

Although going to Stanford would be desirable, I had the proverbial bird in the hand and did not want to gamble on getting the two birds in the bush. I accepted the offer of the CU School of Medicine.

Not long after my interviews with the Stanford and CU medical schools, I returned to the guidance counselor, the one who had urged me to forget about the idea of going to medical school. With a good-natured smile, I handed him two letters—one from Stanford, requesting an interview, and the other from CU, accepting me into medical school.

A look of surprise crossed the guidance counselor's face as he glanced at the letters.

"Congratulations! I'm happy for you, Erica. I want you to know that I thought I had given you good advice." He said he was glad I persevered and sorry he had tried to discourage me. He said he had learned something from me about the power of having a mission to fulfill.

I shook his hand and smiled. After leaving the building, on my walk home I exuberantly belted out the words to Jimmy Cliff's Jamaican reggae song, "You can get it if you really want. You can get it if you really want, but you must try, try and try, try and try, you'll succeed at last...."

Too excited to return to my cramped little room on the edge of campus, I lay down on a grassy area near a huge Douglas fir tree. I looked up at the sky with my arms outstretched to the side and gave thanks to the universe for helping me overcome the many obstacles—including fear and self-doubt—to find my life's purpose as a medical doctor in service to those in need.

One could say that I was born with a genetic predisposition to be a doctor, given my lineage. Yet it took nearly ten years of searching to find something that lay right in front of my nose. What I learned during those ten years was invaluable. As I reviewed the trajectory of my life, I could see that many of my experiences along the way had served to prepare me for my ultimate purpose.

Dr. Samuels had guided me in turning a breakdown into a breakthrough. His therapy helped me become my true self, not the unworthy and never-good-enough person I thought I was. I learned to be self-aware and to have compassion for myself, which in turn led me to have compassion for others. He helped me compost the painful experiences of my childhood—especially with my mother—into a strong desire to help relieve the suffering of others.

My time with the Navajos and Indigenous people of the Andes made it clear to me how much I love to teach and empower my students with useful information in an atmosphere of love and mutual respect.

My mountaineering experiences showed me that I was capable of much more than I realized. The climbing helped me to become strong in mind and body to withstand what might await me on my path.

A stray thought about the Navajo grandmother's prophecy abruptly intruded on my silent musings. I wondered how this prophecy related to my life. Fortunately, I had written in my diary a translated version of what she said in Navajo.

"You are very lucky that the mountain lion came to you. He is your spirit guide. He came to give you his courage, strength, and intense focus because you will need that for what lies ahead." She said I would face many obstacles, some big and life threatening. If I lived through them, I would have a "strong heart and powerful medicine to give to the people."

> *I wonder what those "life-threatening" obstacles could be that I have to overcome to be a good doctor? Was my climb on Aconcagua a life-threatening obstacle? I had a feeling she was talking about even bigger obstacles.*

Letting go of my wandering thoughts, I drifted off to sleep under the Douglas fir tree. I had a dream about working as a doctor in an emergency room treating Navajo patients. The patients smiled in surprise when I spoke to them in their language.

EPILOGUE

You might be wondering what happened to some of the characters who appear in this story. I have been in touch with many of them. As I write this epilogue, I will continue to use their pseudonyms to maintain anonymity.

Although my parents passed from this world long ago, my five siblings are alive and well. The older we get, the tighter our bond with each other has become.

Jean Pierre, my French boyfriend, has stayed in touch with me throughout the years. He and his wife sent their 16-year-old daughter to spend the summer with me in Santa Fe when my son, Barrett, was one year old. Years later, Barrett and I stayed at their home in the countryside outside of Paris, when we were en route to Plum Village to spend our summer with Thich Nhat Hanh, the Vietnamese Buddhist monk.

I have remained in touch with a few of my classmates from high school and college, who have become lifelong friends. Jeff Elliott, my former husband from college days, is still in touch with me. He is happily married with two adult children and continues his photography and artwork. He gave me permission to use his real name in the memoir and said I didn't need his pre-approval for anything I wrote about him.

Pilar, the schoolteacher at La Compañía, found my address and wrote me a long handwritten letter, telling me about her life in Ecuador. Recently, her daughter has also been in touch through email and letters. She said she would like to come to America someday and visit me. Hearing from them brought back a flood of vivid memories.

Arthur and I remained friends and continued to correspond with each other. The last time I saw him in person was at my father's funeral in 1997.

Jorge eventually got over his anger at my betrayal and forgave me. He reached out to me on Facebook about ten years ago, a few months after two of his siblings made contact with me. Jorge is married with three grown children, one of them from his former wife in Hungary. He owns a travel company that mostly operates in the Galápagos Islands, but he will take his clients on other adventures, like to the Himalayas for climbing expeditions. He has urged me to join one of his trips sometime. He said he wants to come visit me in Santa Fe.

Thanks to Facebook, many people from my distant past have contacted me, including people from all the way back to grade school and up through medical school and beyond. A man who happened to find my blog posts had a shock when he realized that I was the same Erica Elliott who taught his freshman orientation course in the Great Smoky Mountains wilderness area in 1976.

After not hearing anything from Mateo for several years, he called my home in Cuba, New Mexico, where I worked in a remote clinic. I have no idea how he found my phone number. He said he had an upcoming training in his field of engineering. The course was at a large hotel in Albuquerque, a 90-minute drive from Cuba. He asked if we could get together at the end of his training on a Sunday.

I drove to Albuquerque to meet Mateo. We both silently cried as we held each other for a long moment. Neither of us brought up our past together in the mountains. It was too painful to dwell on the intensely intimate and meaningful times we had before I left South America. Mateo let me know he was married and had two young daughters, and that he worked as an engineer outside of Quito. After lunch, we took a drive to a nearby wilderness area. The bittersweet mood on our drive was punctured by laughter when Mateo, trying

Epilogue

to practice his English, said in a heavy Spanish accent, "The penises in America are very big and beautiful." Dumbstruck at his words, it took me a minute to realize that he meant to say "the pines." In Spanish, the word for pines is "*pinos.*"

It was painful saying goodbye to Mateo. I knew I would never see him again. My heart ached on the drive home.

The backpacker at the youth hostel in Ushuaia came briefly back into my life 35 years later when my brother, John, a maritime attorney in Seattle, needed to consult with a medical specialist who knew about the kinds of injuries suffered by his client. As John discussed the case with the physician, he noted the pictures of South America on the wall in the doctor's office. John remarked that his sister had served in the Peace Corps in Ecuador in the 1970s and then traveled around the continent. The physician said that in 1976 he had met a woman in the youth hostel in Ushuaia who had worked in the Peace Corps and had climbed to the summit of Aconcagua. John asked if he remembered her name. He answered, "Erica Elliott." A short exchange of emails ensued.

While in Ushuaia, the southernmost city in the world, I looked out over the Beagle channel and made a vow that I would someday go to Antarctica, even though I had no idea how that was going to happen. And 40 years later, I did make a trip to Antarctica, as I had vowed. The trip was a generous gift from an appreciative patient whose three-generational family I had treated medically for over two decades. It was a truly wondrous trip.

Many of my Outward Bound students wrote me letters for several years, telling me how the Outward Bound experience had affected their lives. During a writing retreat in the late 1990s, as we sat in a circle and introduced ourselves, when I said my name, someone on the other side of the circle blurted out, "Oh my god, I thought that was you, Erica. You were my Outward Bound instructor in 1978.

You changed my life." After the retreat was over, she sent me a copy of her journal entries on her course, as well as copies of the photos she took.

Looking back on the journey, I am deeply grateful for all that I learned along the way and for the people I met who profoundly impacted my life.

AFTERWORD

THINKING I HAD REACHED THE FINAL DESTINATION on my path to purpose, I enthusiastically dove headlong into my studies in medical school, followed by a residency in family medicine. Along the way, I gradually began noticing that some aspects of mainstream medicine defied common sense and critical thinking, and they were not in alignment with my values.

I suppressed the little voice inside that had guided my life choices up until then. The little voice said, "This form of medicine is not your path." I paid no attention. Instead, the excitement of being in medical school, along with my competitive nature, propelled me to excel and be a top-notch student.

After ten years of practicing mainstream medicine, disaster struck and derailed my life, just as the Navajo grandmother had prophesized. The disaster served as a portal to the most meaningful life I could have ever imagined.

I will share with you the final episode of the search for purpose in my next memoir.

My first memoir, *Medicine and Miracles in the High Desert: My Life Among the Navajo People*, was published by Bear & Company/Inner Traditions. www.innertraditions.com/books/medicine-and-miracles-in-the-high-desert. It's also available on Amazon and Barnes & Noble.

On my blog site, you will find stories about my life, travels, and useful medical information: www.musingsmemoirandmedicine.com/

ABOUT THE AUTHOR

Erica Elliott lives in Santa Fe, New Mexico, where she has a busy medical practice treating patients from across the country.

After graduating from University of Colorado Medical School and completing her training in family practice, Erica began her medical career in an under-staffed and under-funded health clinic in Cuba, New Mexico. From there, she served in a variety of healthcare settings, including a clinic for indigent care, a busy emergency room, a women's clinic, and a multispecialty clinic.

In 1993, Erica opened her own private practice in her home. Affectionately referred to as "the Health Detective," Erica specializes in diagnosing and treating chronic illnesses by uncovering and addressing the underlying causes. She has given health-related workshops at Esalen and Omega Institute, as well as many other venues.

Erica is a founding member of The Commons, a co-housing community where she raised her son, Barrett Dwyer, and has lived happily since 1993. She gave a TED talk in 2015 about what it was like for her to live in her co-housing community.

Erica blogs about her life and her medical insights at www.musingsmemoirandmedicine.com.